PSYCHIATRY
for the
HOUSE OFFICER

PSYCHIATRY
for the
HOUSE OFFICER

William H. Reid, M.D., M.P.H.

Clinical and Research Psychiatrist, Nebraska Psychiatric
Institute of the University of Nebraska Medical Center and
Assistant Professor of Psychiatry, University of Nebraska
College of Medicine, Omaha
Lecturer in Psychiatry, Northwestern University School of
Medicine, Chicago

 BRUNNER / MAZEL, INC.

Library of Congress Cataloging in Publication Data

Reid, William H   1945–
  Psychiatry for the house officer.

  Bibliography: p.
  Includes index.
  1. Psychiatry—Handbooks, manuals, etc.   2. Crisis intervention (Psy-
chiatry)—Handbooks, manuals, etc.
I. Title. [DNLM: 1. Mental disorders—Handbooks. WM100.3 R35p]
RC457.R45   616.8'9'00202   79–407
ISBN 0–87630–195–2

Published by
BRUNNER/MAZEL, INC.
19 Union Square
New York, NY 10003

MANUFACTURED IN THE UNITED STATES OF AMERICA

To my medical colleagues, and especially Dick R.

Foreword

This is a *Before Book* for house officers and medical student clerks. *Before* a patient's orders are written, *before* an attending is called, or *before* a textbook is consulted, this slim volume can provide a house officer with a brief review and the cogent information needed for the practical management of patients with psychiatric symptoms.

Dr. Reid is to be congratulated for producing a lively, pithy and well-written guide. It will be particularly useful for those house officers and student clerks who are rotating on general medical, surgical, and emergency room services. Its tables on psychotropic medication are well set up for rapid scanning, easily readable, and pertinent. Its sections on Confidentiality, Release of Information, and Legal Aspects of Sexual Problems will aid house officers in approaching these always difficult and potentially explosive problems and in rendering effective, professional and human care.

I predict this book will become a companion of the reflex hammers, stethoscopes, and blood drawing tubes that reside in the pockets of many white coats, or will be found among other tools in the house officers' bags.

K. H. Blacker, M.D.
*Associate Dean for
Hospital Educational Affairs,
University of California
School of Medicine, Davis*

Introduction

This small addition to the burgeoning literature of medicine is designed for only one purpose: usefulness. To this end, a psychiatrist experienced in both the practice and teaching of the specialty has combined his efforts with those of a number of other clinicians, including a senior house officer in family practice. Field trials with groups of practicing physicians, house officers and medical students preceded final revisions of the text.

We emphasize without apology that this book is not a complete treatment of medical psychiatry. Instead, this is a brief handbook, designed for use when time is short and the reader requires a concise, practical summary of psychiatry as it presents in nonpsychiatric practice and as it interfaces with the rest of medicine. Sources of more complete information are listed. The author recommends their use and suggests that they, or other references, be consulted before definitive diagnosis is made and treatment continued. In addition, most communities and institutions have available psychiatrists who welcome the opportunity to consult with their colleagues in the service of the patient and of communication among medical practitioners.

Psychiatry is a science and a medical specialty. It is also an art in the best clinical tradition. We have attempted to represent both of these important aspects of work with patients—that is, to paraphrase and outline the crux of medically relevant information, yet to address our art with the understanding it deserves.

Finally, a tenet from all of medicine: *Listen to the patient!* He or she has the information you need in order to make the essential decisions and is often trying to share that information with you.

W.H.R.

Acknowledgments

Dr. Kent Myers generously shared with the author his experience and suggestions from the viewpoint of both house officer and family practitioner. Also gratefully acknowledged is the assistance of Drs. Helen Morrison and Alfred P. French in the preparation of the sections on Children and on Couple and Family Therapy. Dr. David K. Kentsmith gave valuable advice for the section on Sexual Dysfunction. Drafts and the final manuscript were ably prepared by Marilyn Pittillo. Finally, our thanks to the many students, house officers and practitioners who reviewed, used and commented upon earlier drafts of this work.

Contents

PSYCHIATRY
for the
HOUSE OFFICER

I History and Mental Status Examination

I.A: HISTORY

The psychiatric history is the most important single factor in arriving at an accurate diagnosis and formulating a plan for treatment. A complete history is neither intrusive nor embarrassing to the patient any more than is a complete medical history. When done professionally and attentively, it can be a beginning for the therapeutic relationship. The format shown on pp. 6–7 is one that works well in most situations. It supplies most needed information and can be completed in 30–45 minutes.

The following are some brief explanations of items on the history format example, in order of their appearance on the form:

Past forms of treatment and their success (or failure) are not only helpful in choosing among present treatment choices; they may give clues as to diagnoses made in the past. For example, if a patient states that he was treated for "nerves" but that he received "Prolixin shots," then one should suspect that the previous episode had to do with a serious psychosis.

Appetite, sleeping patterns, and history of *crying spells* or *suicidal behavior* are important primarily in evaluating dimensions of depression.

The *medical history* may be brief but should be as thorough as is indicated under the circumstances. Knowing the primary or family physician allows important communication, both now, when you need his impressions of the patient, and later, when you will share hospital course and discharge plans with him or her.

1

Serious *childhood illness* which involved physical or emotional separation from the parents at any age is important to document, as is any history of birth trauma or perinatal distress.

The *family history* and family dynamics may be vital to the diagnosis. These may include family histories of mental illness, familial medical illness, responses to psychotropic medications, suicidal histories, traditional ways in which the family deals with its problems, etc. A knowledge of family size, stability, birth order and timing of siblings, and marital history are all helpful.

Social history and "premorbid" characteristics as detailed on the history form should evoke a chronology of the patient's life which will summon up a mental picture of him or her (although not a stereotype based upon incomplete information).

I.B: MENTAL STATUS EXAMINATION

This section is designed to explain and augment the items on the history and examination form (pp. 6–7) in order of appearance on the form.

First, is there evidence from the history or early interview that medical evaluation is needed? Physical examination should be part of the complete mental status examination, although in some cases it may be limited or may be performed by some physician other than the psychotherapist.

Your first sight of the patient is the start of the examination. Is he alone or with someone? Does the companion remain in the room? Where is the patient interviewed? Where does he choose to sit?

What is his physical *appearance:* Condition of body, dress, grooming?

Are his *demeanor* and level of *activity* during the interview appropriate? Does he react appropriately toward you? Or is he avoiding, aggressive, or meek? Does he meet your gaze when appropriate? More than is appropriate?

Is his *affect* or *facial expression* appropriate to the current situation? Does it reflect the situation as the patient perceives it (e.g., if he has delusions of someone trying to hurt him, does he seem fearful)? Is the face normally animated, or "flat"? Does his *mood* indicate sadness? Anger? Anxiety? How does his body positioning or posture reflect (or contrast with) his mood? Is he *labile,* shifting rapidly from one affect to another (e.g., crying) without much outside stimulus to do so (often a sign of organic CNS deficit)?

How does the patient *communicate* with you? Communication is the most consistent indication of the patient's *thought process.* Is it verbal? Wholly nonverbal? Appropriate to the situation? Appropriate to his perception of the situation? Is it logical and connected, or is it disconnected ("loose")? How loose (e.g., almost understandable, or seemingly random)?

What of his *thought content,* as measured by his communication (it is risky to try to infer the content of someone's thoughts when he is not verbalizing to you)? Is he misperceiving sensory input (*illusion*), perhaps basing it on an unshakable set of beliefs that are inconsistent with reality (*delusion*)? Does he perceive sensory input when none is apparent (*hallucination*)? Are these hallucinations auditory? Visual? Olfactory? Tactile? Gustatory? Are they pleasant? Frightening? Repulsive? Are they organized and understandable within the context of the patient's frame of reference, or are they more vague, perhaps seemingly unrelated to anything?

The above symptoms indicate the extent of the patient's *contact with reality.* Is he able to ask himself what is real and what is not (*reality testing*)? Is he concerned that he may be losing contact with reality? What measures does he take to retain contact with reality?

Are there signs of *depression* (posture, facies, voice quality, crying) or of *anxiety* (posture, facies, perspiration, physical activity)? Are there areas in the interview that the patient skips over, either by accident or through purposeful avoidance? Does he sometimes pause before responding to certain lines of inquiry? Does he seem to forget or "block" simple information that should be accessible?

Take a few moments to go through a brief examination for possible signs of *organic CNS deficit.* Be thorough, even though some portions of this examination may seem obvious. Occasionally, a patient who jokes about the "silliness" or obvious nature of a question may be avoiding the fact that it is difficult for him to answer it.

1. Check *orientation,* including person, place, complete date (including the year!) and situation. Note sensorium.
2. Test *memory* in three modes:
   a. *reflex* (ability to immediately repeat a series of words or numbers);
   b. *recent* (ability to remember three unrelated words for several minutes, once they have been clearly understood as a memory test and given in the language of the patient's choice, and to say them back to you); and
   c. *remote* (ability to recall events of several hours to several years past). Do not test memory with "What did you have for breakfast?" unless you know what the patient had for breakfast.
3. Test *judgment* (not just an organic function) with appropriate hypothetical situations ("What would you do if . . . ?") and try to get some impression of capacity for *abstract thought* (as opposed to "concreteness" of thought and conceptualization) via conversation or perhaps common proverbs. The "concrete" patient may respond to "People who live in glass houses . . ." with, "Someone's liable to throw rocks back and break the windows"; the CNS impaired patient perhaps with, "It would break the windows"; and the patient with good abstract thought with, "A critical person often has flaws of his own."
4. *Cognition* is somewhat addressed above but should also be tested with regard to arithmetic and intellectual ability, bearing in mind the patient's background and education. General information and general intelligence may be addressed by asking about such things as current events, the names of past Presidents, etc.

5. Shallowness or lability of *affect* (see above) may signify organic deficit.
6. Finally, a few simple neurological tests such as those for agnosia, anomia, dyslexia, agraphia, cerebellar function, cranial nerves, and the like will occasionally be productive and warrant the few minutes that they require.

Confidentiality

Information gained from the patient should not be shared with anyone except the treating staff, and that only on a need-to-know basis, unless you have good reason to believe that withholding information may seriously endanger the patient or another individual. Legally speaking, in most jurisdictions written information in a patient's chart is subject to anonymous review by a number of boards and agencies, and to subpoena in civil and criminal proceedings. In addition, the patient generally has a legal right to inspect his chart unless the physician can rapidly and conclusively show that information in it is likely to be harmful to the patient. In short, you must find a compromise between the vital need to document and communicate information via the chart, and the potential harm that may come to the patient (and to his current and future therapeutic relationships) as a result of the written word.

Release of Information

You will frequently be asked about the patient's condition, whether he can work, whether he can be trusted, whether he can drive, etc. The ethical and legal principles of release of information vary only slightly from state to state, and apply not only to outside individuals and agencies but to the patient's relatives as well. With regard to insurance companies, a carefully explained and firmly presented policy of minimal information (e.g., identifying data, diagnosis, and general treatment measures taken) is usually acceptable even to companies who initially may request a large amount of personal information. The data that the company are likely to request, as well as

PSYCHIATRIC HISTORY AND EXAMINATION FORM
(See Text for Explanations)

Name_____ Aliases _____

Age___ D.O.B._____ Soc. Sec. No._____ Marital Status___ Date_____

Address_____ Telephone_____

Relative/Close Friend for Contact_____

Source of Hx (Patient, Relative, etc.)_____

Ethnic Background_____ Native or Preferred Language_____

— —

Presenting Complaint (in patient's words)_____

_____

Source and Method of Psychiatric Referral_____

Hx of Present Complaint; Past Rx?; Was Past Rx Successful?_____

_____

Current and Past Psych Meds; Successful? Allergies or Med Reactions?_____

_____

Other Psych Hx, including Hospitalizations and Therapy_____

_____

Appetite/Weight Loss_____ Sleep Patterns_____

Crying Spells_____ Suicidal Thoughts/Attempts_____

— —

Medical Hx: Family Physician_____

Current Illnesses, Meds, Treatments, Allergies_____

_____

Childhood Illnesses, Surgeries, Hospitalizations_____

_____

Adult Med Hx, Menstrual Hx, System Review_____

_____

— —

Family Hx: Health (or Time and Cause of Death) and Description of Parents, Siblings, Children_____

_____

Marital Hx and Description of Spouse (or other persons living with Patient)

_____

Hx of Mental Illness, Mental Hospitalizations, Suicidal Behavior, or Alcohol Abuse in any Close Relative (Parents, Siblings, Grandparents, Aunts, Uncles, or Cousins)_____

_____

PSYCHIATRIC HISTORY AND EXAMINATION FORM
(continued)

_ _

Social Hx: Occupation/Work Environment_____

    Education_____ Tobacco/Caffeine/Diet_____

    Interests/Activities/Daily Lifestyle—_____

    Description of Current Household_____

    Brief Description of Childhood, School, Adolescence, Military Experience, Job Experience_____

    Alcohol, Drug, and Legal Hx_____

    Sexual Hx (Detailed or not, as appropriate)_____

_ _

MENTAL STATUS EXAMINATION: (See Text for Detailed Explanation)

    Presenting Setting_____ Seen Alone?____

    Physical and Personal Appearance _____

    Demeanor and Activity in Interview_____

    Affect/Mood/Facial and Body Expression_____

    Communication/Process of Thought and Speech_____

    Content of Thought and Speech/Delusions/Hallucinations_____

    Contact with Reality_____

    Signs of Depression/Anxiety_____

    Organic Signs (Judgment, Orientation, Memory, Cognition)_____

_ _

IMPRESSIONS: Differential Dx._____

    Is further medical or psych workup indicated?_____

your policy for release of information for purposes of reimbursement, should be clearly explained to the patient as early as possible in the treatment. In every other instance of request for information, a conservative approach is recommended. If your institution has a special policy regarding psychiatric records, use it. If not, you may wish to follow our routine of requiring that each request for information be accompanied by a signed, witnessed, recently dated authorization from the patient which specifies the type of information to be released and the particular parties who are to receive it. Most psychiatric patients are legally (and actually) competent to understand and give such a release. Even if you feel that the patient is acting unwisely, if he or she has not been adjudged legally incompetent, the physician should not, in general, obstruct the patient's right to access to and disposition of information about himself.

Note the age of majority in your state as it applies to release of information. Children old enough to understand the information should be included in the release. Even if their consent is not legally "required," it is in their best interest to understand and participate in such actions. Finally, when releasing information, note in the record that you are doing so in good faith, that so far as you know the information is legally accessible, and that it is to be used toward the best interests of the patient.

II Presentations

This section deals with what the physician first sees, and the point at which his or her thinking must begin.

II.A: EMERGENCIES

1. Suicide

The main principle of acute suicide prevention is not to permanently cure the patient or alleviate the precipitating condition, but *to alleviate the present discomfort and pressure in order to allow time for consideration of other ways to deal with the problems at hand.* Suicidal behavior may be divided into "completed acts" and "threatened acts." Both must be taken seriously, even if they appear nonlethal or designed to attract attention, since

    a. the odds of survival may be good but the stakes are very high;
    b. you do not know the whole story unless you have worked closely with the patient for years; and
    c. the patient's idea of "serious" threats or attempts may be quite different from that of a physician.

The patient is in trouble and pain, even if you feel he/she is at low risk.

Completed Acts:

    a. Assess medical needs.
    b. Don't try to counsel somnolent or intoxicated patients but do support, reassure and see that they get humane treatment.

c. Don't attempt to treat over the telephone. Give emergency first-aid instructions and try to get the patient to the hospital rather than taking the chance of misjudging lethality and slighting the patient.

d. Offer counseling and follow-up.

Differentiating between a "gesture" and an "attempt" involves careful assessment; it should be done by qualified professionals, if at all.

Threatened Acts:

a. Take seriously and offer support, time, and in-person contact.

b. Be warm and supportive, but honest and straightforward in all communication.

c. Convey the impression that you know the patient is troubled and in pain.

d. Help the patient consider the consequences of attempted or completed suicide on those around him and important to him (including himself).

e. Explore other means by which the patient might express or deal with the feelings that he sees as making it necessary to attempt suicide (sadness, depression, loss [see II. B below], anger, rejection, and uselessness).

f. *Never* "dare" a patient to kill himself by playing down the attempt, by being punitive, or by showing him how to do it ("If you really wanted to kill yourself you'd cut here on your carotid instead of your wrists").

g. Don't use theatrical methods in suicide counseling. These are best reserved for therapists who don't know any better.

h. Once you are convinced of the seriousness and/or lethality of a threat, do not hesitate at serious treatment measures, including legal commitment. At that point, do not allow yourself to be talked out of hospitalization, etc., by the patient, who may promise, cajole, embarrass or even threaten in order to avoid good, conservative treatment.

Although one should not rely upon methods of prediction of lethality, the following are associated with increased risk of serious attempt or death:

a. *previous attempts,* even if of low lethality;
b. *loss* of spouse or significant other person (including by divorce); loss of one's feeling of usefulness, of feelings of attractiveness, youth, health, self-esteem; loss of hope (*hopelessness*);
c. *pain,* which may be physical or emotional, and may be related to depression, loss, or hopelessness, as above;
d. *psychosis*—the patient who is out of contact with reality is
    i. less predictable;
    ii. less aware of the lethality of his attempt;
    iii. less able to control the lethality of his attempt.
e. *Plan*—the existence of a plan for suicide means greater risks of completion.

The patient's idea of serious loss or pain may be different from your own. When confronted with a patient who is not presenting as suicidal but who shows some of the above signs, or has vague complaints or a feeling of "saying good-bye," consider suicidal dangers and ask the patient about it. Don't worry about putting ideas into his head; if he is self-destructive, the ideas are already there and need desperately to be discovered.

Never underestimate the suicidal potential of people just be-cause they are well-educated or professionals. Ask, especially when loss or threat of loss is apparent (e.g., in the public figure who has been arrested or the physician who has been caught abusing drugs).

2. Severe Agitation

Agitation becomes an emergency when it begins to endanger the patient or someone around him. Acute agitation may be related to emotional or organic causes, but most situations fall into a few, sometimes overlapping, categories important to formulation and treatment:

a. *Confusion* about what is going on may be related to "fight-or-flight" reaction after trauma, dulling of senses by medications or other intoxicants, sensory deprivation (sometimes iatrogenic), etc., such that the patient cannot be expected to have any understanding that he should be calm. *Treatment:* "Talking down," reinstituting sensory communication in all five senses, explaining what is going on, and a non-assaultive manner on the part of yourself and staff.

b. *Misperceived Attack,* a patient's fear of assault or belief that he is being attacked, may often be attributed to psychosis or intoxication. However, much of what we do in hospitals is (hopefully benevolent) assault upon the patient's body. Partially conscious, post-ictal, post-traumatic, post-MI, sedated, intoxicated, unsophisticated, elderly, or CVA patients may misread efforts to treat, perform diagnostic procedures, or protect (e.g., via confining belts and siderails) and react defensively. *Treatment:* as above, explanation of procedures, removal of constraints as soon as possible, attempts to find avenues of communication.

Medical Treatment: When rapid calming is essential and the patient's emotional comfort and well-being must take a back seat to medical emergency or danger to others, use drugs whose primary action is short-term sedation (short-acting barbiturates, IM benzodiazepines such as diazepam) and consider the effects of such drugs' actions and metabolism on any medical problem involved (see Chapter III on *Medications*). Unless the patient is known to have a psychiatric disorder for which neuroleptics (chlorpromazine, haloperidol, etc.; see *Medications*) are appropriate, do not use them to calm agitation. Such drugs have long action, may further reduce sensory input, and may cloud the diagnostic picture with sedation or iatrogenic confusional syndromes.

Aggressive and/or psychotic patients who are more purposeful in their agitated acts may respond to a quiet but firm "show of force." The physician may see the patient in the company of several aides who do not directly threaten the patient but who make it clear that the doctor is in control and that the patient will not be allowed to harm anyone, including himself. Such a patient may ask why so many people are present or accuse the doctor of being afraid. He is usually relieved when it is explained that although he is indeed frightening, the staff on hand can deal with his feelings and actions and will not allow any damage to be done.

Finally, if there is serious danger to staff or others, the patient's emotional comfort must come second to public safety. Only a foolish physician would expose himself or others to danger by "playing hero," trying to disarm a patient, or otherwise attempting to operate outside our familiar element of the helping professions. In such a situation, call for lots of help, including perhaps the police. The police are the community's experts in handling dangerous situations and protecting people; they have the better chance of doing the least harmful thing for all concerned.

First, protect yourself and those around you.

3. Acute Anxiety/Panic

Acute anxiety:

   a. is basically (but not always exactly) *fear;*
   b. may lead to agitation (section 2 above);
   c. hurts, and makes the patient feel that things are intolerable for him.

Treatment (see also Chapter on *Psychotropic Medications*) involves:

   a. Calmness and a quiet, strong appearance in the physician or therapist;
   b. Acceptance of the fact that the patient is hurting, perhaps with platonic touching (e.g., a hand on the shoulder);

c. Anxiolytic—not antipsychotic—medication (see Chapter III), although it may
   i. dull the sensorium and prevent needed alertness,
   ii. "cheat" the patient out of a necessary emotional experience (see II.B:3 *Grief,* for example) which will be even harder to deal with when it resurfaces at some later date, and
   iii. lead to dependence upon pharmacologic or other outside supports for dealing with less-than-urgent situations.
d. Patients with repeated attacks of severe anxiety should receive an opportunity for nonpharmacologic management (e.g., psychotherapy).

4. Acute Mania

This is an acute manifestation of an affective psychosis discussed later in the text (pp. 21–22).

a. Frenzied *activity,* which the patient cannot stop, is apparent: moving, talking; thoughts may pour rapidly and disconnectedly out of his mouth (cf., the toad in the novel *Wind in the Willows*).
b. The history may include similar episodes, grandiosity, hypersexuality, poor judgment (especially financial), and little or no sleep (but no fatigue).
c. Sleep deprivation may be an early manifestation and may trigger the acute hyperactivity.
d. *Differential diagnosis* includes other sources of sleep deprivation and some drug abuses and reactions (stimulants, hallucinogens, others).
e. There is considerable danger of fatigue and taxing of body functions, especially in patients with concomitant organic illness.

Treatment:
a. Rapid cessation of hyperactivity, by any means possible, is necessary.
b. High doses of medication may be required.

c. If the diagnosis is clear, give haloperidol 5–10 mg. IM per 30–60 minutes, up to 60 mg. in 12 hours *or* high doses of sedative phenothiazines (e.g., up to a gram or more of chlorpromazine in graded doses), with observation for hypotension, hyperthermia, decreased fluid intake, and other side effects. See *Rapid Tranquilization* (pp. 52–53).

d. Hospitalize for observation and definitive treatment.

5. Dystonias/Other Acute Side Effects of Psychiatric Medications

Most side effects of psychiatric medications are self-limiting, with very little morbidity or mortality. (See also Chapter III on *Psychotropic Medications*).

Dystonias: Acute muscle spasm, often of the trunk, back or neck muscles, and sometimes involving ocular musculature ("oculogyric crisis"). May be quite painful, twisting the body about, and is usually very frightening. *History* includes recent intake of routine or higher than usual (in the case of a patient who has been taking the medication for some time) doses of neuroleptic meds (phenothiazines, haloperidol, thioxanthenes), usually in young adult patients. Sometimes associated with noncompliance with prescription for antiparkinsonian medication. *Treatment* is rapidly-acting and diagnostic:

a. IM or IV benztropine (Cogentin) 2–6 mg. (expect anticholinergic side effects). Symptoms will decrease in moments with IV route. If no clear alleviation after 6–8 mg., strongly suspect another disease process.

b. Maintain improvement on oral benztropine or other synthetic antiparkinsonian (e.g., trihexyphenidyl [Artane, Tremin], 4–10 mg. per day) and reassure patient.

c. Follow-up appointment with psychiatrist to adjust meds.

d. Patient may discontinue the antipsychotic medication until it is re-evaluated; however, do not tell him he shouldn't be taking the drug or that he is "allergic" to it, since he may need the medication badly and proper adjustment may eliminate major side effects.

Other Non-Rare Acute
Adverse Reactions: *Treatment* (see Chapter III):

a. *Heatstroke, altered body temperature control* with antipsychotic meds.

    –Medical Rx for hyperpyrexia. Prevention: avoid high temperatures, saunas, hot sun.

b. *Hypotension,* especially orthostatic, with antipsychotics (especially IM) and antidepressants.

    –*Avoid epinephrine.* Lower med doses; caution concerning body position, high temp. Tolerance usually develops. Levarterenol if severe.

c. *Hepatic compromise.*

    –Prevention: Note that all current antipsychotics and antidepressants are livertoxic except lithium.

d. *Acute electrolyte imbalance* in patients taking lithium carbonate.

    –Prevention: Maintain adequate salt and fluid intake; watch for concurrent causes of diarrhea or vomiting. Watch for ECG changes. Reestablish balance.

e. *Cardiac arrythmias* with lithium, antidepressants, some antipsychotics, especially in predisposed patients.

    –Rule out MI. Lower dosage, switch to a less cardiotoxic med.

f. *Acute psychosis* in patients taking stimulants or antiparkinsonian meds.

    –Lower dosage of antiparkinsonian; discontinue stimulant. Suspect overdosage or abuse in either case.

6. Intoxications

a. Evaluate medical needs, especially before giving drugs which may act upon or be metabolized through already compromised body systems (e.g., additive CNS depressant

effects *or* metabolism of a calmative through the over-
loaded liver of an alcoholic).
b. Most common nonmedical problems involve agitation
and/or panic.
c. Treat as noted above for these symptoms (II. A: 2, 3).
d. Hallucinogen abuse syndromes are best treated with quiet
surroundings and someone available to sit with the patient. Anxiolytics such as diazepam IM may be useful. Do
not use neuroleptics (phenothiazines, haloperidol).
e. In differentiating hallucinogen intoxication from emotional causes of psychotic symptoms, wait several hours or
even days before using the "schizophrenic" or "manic-
depressive" label, since this is a serious and lasting
diagnosis.
f. Amphetamines, even in routine doses, can produce symptoms indistinguishable from paranoid schizophrenia.

**Acute medical needs, as well as potential medical or iatro-
genic sources for apparent simple "intoxication," must be
explored early in the evaluation. The history is crucial.**

For situations of *overdose,* see below; for *withdrawal* situations, see pp. 35–42.

7. Overdoses

Medical management of the overdose should be instituted as
necessary (see *Drug Abuse* and *Bibliography* sections). Acute
anticholinergic syndromes, e.g., from overdose of neuroleptics,
antidepressants, or antiparkinsonian drugs, may be reversed
with physostigmine, 1–4 mg. IM or slow IV. Repeat as needed.

As mentioned before, psychotherapeutic intervention is not
useful until the patient is fully awake and alert. It is inappropriate to refer for psychiatric evaluation a patient who is
acutely intoxicated or somnolent.

The patient who has taken an overdose may not be in a life-
threatening situation, may have gotten the physician-on-call out
of a sound sleep, and/or may be keeping you from more productive work elsewhere, HOWEVER:

Don't take your anger out on the patient and don't tolerate cruelty to the patient by other members of the staff. It is the patient who is in the most trouble and pain and who probably has the least ability to cope with it.

8. Medical Emergencies Masking as Psychiatric Symptoms

Symptom/ Sign	Watch For:	Possible Hints
Psychosis; Psychotic behavior	Any of a number of problems, including CNS lesions, hemodynamic causes, hematologic imbalance, infection, toxins (liver, kidney, muscle, other), intoxications, environmental or sensory deprivations, iatrogenic causes.	Confusion or altered consciousness; first psychotic episode, especially in persons over 30; pre-existing medical illness or prescription for same.
Depression	Many diseases, especially those with a deteriorating process or which produce fatigue; iatrogenic causes (especially medications); substance abuse.	First episode; especially in older person; associated early CNS signs; decreased alertness; confusion; known medical illness or prescription.
Confusion; Confused agitation	Organic delirium; iatrogenic causes; CNS hemodynamics; alcohol/barbiturate/etc., withdrawal; ictal/post-ictal states; sensory or environmental deprivation; electrolyte imbalance.	*Any confusion or disorientation is organic until proved otherwise.*

"Functional" disability; "Hysterical" symptoms or paralysis	Be sure of your diagnosis of "functional" or "hysterical."	First episode; no prior similar history; no obvious "secondary gain."
Drug or alcohol intoxication	Underlying severe addiction; medical complications of same.	History; needle tracks; nutritional status; early withdrawal signs.

First priority diagnostic measures to accompany history and physical exam:

a. Blood sugar   d. Serum electrolytes   g. Toxicology
b. Blood gasses   e. Electrocardiogram
c. BUN   f. CBC

Avoid unnecessary sedation.

Remember: Psychiatric disease, hypochondria, hysterical symptoms and the like do not confer upon the patient any immunity against ordinary organic illness or injury.

II.B: DEPRESSION

There are four basic tenets about depression to keep in mind:

a. Depression is very *common;*
b. It can present in a variety of seemingly unrelated ways (see below);
c. It is among the most painful of diseases; and
d. It is often treatable with a high rate of success.

Depression is most accurately seen on a continuum or "spectrum," rather than as a group of discrete syndromes; however, the following separations are made in order to clarify treatment issues.

1. Situational/"Exogenous" Depression

This is a depression which seems primarily related to events located outside the psyche (e.g., environment, physical illness). It has in the past been termed "exogenous" or "reactive."

a. Patient can often recognize the fact that he or she is depressed (sad, blue, down) and discuss it.
b. Patient can present with subtly destructive living patterns or with extra activity (e.g., drug abuse, extramarital affairs, denial of physical or medical limitations).
c. Classic symptoms/signs include:
    i. sad or depressed feelings, hopelessness, helplessness;
    ii. loss of interest, feelings of apathy, ennui;
    iii. altered work or school performance;
    iv. *changes* in appetite, sexual habits, amount of sleep;
    v. changes in pattern of sleep (e.g., early awakening, insomnia);
    vi. fatigue;
    vii. increased complaints of physical symptoms;
    viii. increased demands for the doctor's attention.

When any of these, and especially more than one, are encountered, one should suspect depression, even if denied by the patient.

Treatment of situational depression with supportive counseling or psychotherapy, environmental manipulation, encouragement of activity, and passage of time is more likely to be successful than "antidepressant" medications. Anti-anxiety meds may be used at times, but these are aimed only at anxiety, not at the depression itself (see *Medications* section). Sometimes anti-anxiety meds (anxiolytics) may remove protective anxiety and make the underlying depression more symptomatic.

In the case of situational depression, a great deal of good may be done by letting the patient know you understand he is in pain, and that depression of this type is almost always self-limiting:

a. You know it hurts and seems hopeless now, but
b. you are optimistic that he will feel better with time.

2. Severe/"Endogenous" Depression

A less common but more malignant form of depression is that which seems to come primarily from within the psyche; hence the still-used term "endogenous":

a. Deep feelings of self-deprecation, hopelessness, helplessness in the face of ordinary living.

b. There may be external factors which make things worse or bring out an underlying potential for depression, but these external influences are secondary in importance.

c. Many of the above symptoms of situational depression may be present, perhaps many or all of them at the same time.

d. *Vegetative* signs are frequent; i.e., physiological alterations such as constipation, anorexia and weight loss, slowing of physical movements (psychomotor retardation).

e. Severe depression is more frequent in mid- to late-life than before age 30.

f. Serious depressive syndromes include:

   i. "involutional" depressions, which are related to a turning inward of feelings after a major life change or loss (e.g., menopause);

   ii. some major post-partum depressions;

   iii. severe depression of the elderly and late middle aged;

   iv. other "affective psychoses," some of which may alternate with manic-appearing states ("bipolar" affective illness); and

   v. some special childhood and infant syndromes (e.g., "anaclitic" depression).

These depressions are far more prone than less severe ones to:

a. lead to serious suicide attempts;

b. decompensate into psychosis (loss of contact with reality), which may look either stereotypically depressive or "agitated"; and

c. *not* abate with time or with psychotherapy alone.

Treatment of severe depression, once diagnosis is made, is straightforward and usually effective. Treatment

a. often involves antidepressant medication (see *Medication* section) *or* (usually not "and")
b. electroconvulsive therapy (see Chapter IV on *Other Organic Therapies*);
c. must be vigorous, closely monitored, and *of sufficient length and dosage* (e.g., several months or even years at 150+ mg. of imipramine) to prevent return of symptoms after discontinuation;
d. may involve hospitalization;
e. may include measures for environmental manipulation, social support, etc.;
f. may involve an acceptable outlet for anger or other emotions (e.g., "non-productive" hobbies).

Suicide (see *Suicide* section, page 9): Watch for signs of worsening depression and suicide risk.

Be alert to the possibility that with apparent improvement and increased energy level <u>the patient may gain the ability to plan and carry out a suicide attempt.</u> Many suicides occur within a few weeks of the first signs of clinical and physical improvement, just when the physician and family have begun to relax their vigilance. Discuss suicide with the patient and his family.

3. Grief/Bereavement

Grief resembles depression but is different in a number of important ways:

a. It is a natural and universal response to acute loss of any kind.
b. Such loss includes, but is not limited to, death of loved ones or one's own illness or dying.
c. Grief is *dynamic,* with a usually predictable path and a purpose which is related to growth and adaptation.

d. It is painful, but ordinarily does not require active medical intervention.

e. It is normally limited to several months' duration.

Inappropriate intervention in the natural grief process may be detrimental.

Treatment of severe loss or death of a loved one involves the realization that in most cases the appropriate treatment is to allow an environment in which natural processes can do their work:

a. Avoid emotion-dulling medications.

b. Do not attempt to "protect" a surviving spouse or child by keeping him or her away from the facts of death.

c. Encourage everyone's attendance at the funeral, even (and especially) children and aged relatives.

d. Teach the family the difference between "support" for each other and ill-advised "protection." Recommend against "sending the kids away for awhile" or "having all Dad's things put away before Mom gets home."

Mother must herself put away Dad's things, and with them each memory and tear. Children must have this last opportunity at the funeral to experience the realness of the deceased parent(s), lest the last memory they have is of a cruel wresting away without any chance to go through their strong feelings. Each person must figuratively—and eventually permanently—bury the lost love object.

Occasionally, often as a result of the well-meant mistakes cited above, grief work is incompletely or improperly accomplished. This may result in lasting symptoms or in an "arrest" of the process, with resurfacing of symptoms at some future time. When diagnosed, such aberrant grief reactions have a good prognosis with relatively brief psychotherapeutic treatment.

Delayed or aberrant grief reaction should be considered in the differential diagnosis of new depression or psychosis, and a history of past losses examined.

II.C: ANXIETY/FEAR

For our purposes, these are identical. The body is being made aware of some perceived threat to its integrity and must prepare either to fight or to run. Since physical survival is usually not an issue in our society, many of these emotional and physiological responses may seem on the surface useless or illogical. The source of much of the threat may be unconscious psychological conflict, which means that the discomfort is much harder to dissipate through the ancient methods of "fight or flight." In addition, if one's usual channels of protection—either physical or emotional—from anxiety-producing situations are blocked, the symptoms may increase dramatically.

1. Situational Anxiety

This type of anxiety is a response to real, identifiable external stresses; therefore, it is "logical," if only to the patient. It may arise from:

a. fear of death pending surgery;
b. concerns over a painless but unfamiliar diagnostic procedure;
c. worry that one will be caught unprepared during a class or seminar;
d. worry about losing one's job.

Treatment may include:

a. education about the true nature of the environment or stress;
b. understanding or support during a difficult time;
c. mild anxiolytic medication (see *Medication* section).

2. Neurotic Anxiety

This type of anxiety:

a. may be similar to, or participate in, situational anxiety;
b. has exactly the same potential physiological components

(perspiration, gastrointestinal symptoms, tachycardia, tremor, hyperpnea, etc.);

c. has causes which are hidden in the patient's psyche but may show themselves "symbolically" in symptoms or behaviors;

d. may be kept in good control by such behaviors or "neurotic" defenses and not present as a problem for the patient; *or*

e. may, from stresses internal or external to the patient, surface and require treatment.

Treatment is as follows:

a. symptomatic treatment as for Situational Anxiety, above, in order to restore the patient's own balance of defenses or to support him until the passage of extraordinary stress (see cautions under *Grief/Bereavement,* pp. 22–23);

b. psychotherapy to examine the unseen components of the overt symptoms (see Chapter V on *Psychotherapies*).

II.D: PSYCHOTIC BEHAVIOR

There are many situations in which both normal and psychiatrically disordered people may show or experience psychotic or "crazy" behavior. We shall define the existence of psychosis from a phenomenologic or observational point of view. It refers to *grossly inappropriate thinking and/or behavior which do not seem related to the environment or situation as we perceive it, and which are so out of step with it that one might refer to a "loss of touch with reality."* It is often, although not always, such that it makes sense to the patient in his emotional perception of things; however, we make the judgment that it is severely inappropriate to a "reasonable man's" concept of reality.

1. Organic Psychosis

Any psychosis, especially a first psychotic episode or one occurring past the age of 30, should be medically explored.

Hints of the organic nature of psychotic symptoms can be gotten from the history and a brief mental status exam (see *History and Examination; Agitation,* and *Medical Emergencies Masking as Psychiatric Symptoms* sections).

Treatment is based upon treatment of the underlying organic pathology. Symptomatic relief is associated with the following:

a. Generally avoid "antipsychotic" drugs such as phenothiazines and butyrophenones, except as noted in *Medication* section.

b. First attempts at treatment should aim at orientation and unclouding of sensorium:

   i. verbal orientation, place, date, etc.;

   ii. allowing quiet visitors whenever possible;

   iii. introducing familiar objects into the hospital or nursing home setting;

   iv. patient explanation of all activities, procedures, instruments, etc.;

   v. minimizing disorienting or sedating medications; and

   vi. allowing human contact with staff (e.g., in an ICU).

c. If above fails, consider mild antianxiety medications but:

   i. start with low doses;

   ii. monitor increases in dosage or changes in regimen closely; and

   iii. treat worsening symptoms first with a *decrease* in medication rather than with escalation of intervention (see *Medication* section).

d. Antisenility meds, cerebral vasodilators, etc., have little or no proved effectiveness.

e. Remember that many confused or even somnolent patients can still hear and often understand conversation; therefore:

   i. Speaking to the patient who cannot respond may be very helpful in the long run.

   ii. Take care that staff does not carelessly carry on conversations which may be unsettling.

Since organically-based inappropriateness is often related to hematologic, toxic, or electrical compromise of CNS

tissue, neuroleptic ("antipsychotic") agents, which are CNS-toxic, should generally be avoided.

The all-too-familiar cycle of

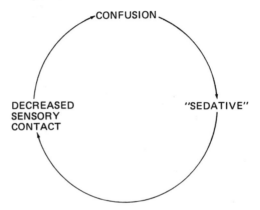

in the elderly patient
is too often played out with gerotoxic drugs, with an end result óf severe compromise or even obtundation misdiagnosed as being secondary to chronic or acute vascular disease.

2. Functional Psychosis

This type of psychosis is unrelated to gross medical illness. It may be discussed in three categories:

a. *Crisis reactions:*
   i. are situational, usually self-limiting;
   ii. are often treatable with either psychotherapeutic or pharmacologic approaches;
   iii. may include severe grief reactions and reactions to sensory deprivation (e.g., in hospital ICU's) or incarceration (not malingering);
   iv. *do not indicate chronic mental illness.*
   v. Once the crisis-related diagnosis is made, the patient and family can be reassured and effective treatment instituted (see *Medication* and other specific treatment sections).

b. Psychotic episodes *related to underlying nonpsychotic emotional disease:*

i. may be seen as temporary setbacks within serious neurotic or characterologic processes.

ii. The underlying nonpsychotic process ordinarily does not require the patient to drastically alter his perception of reality, but it may fail under stress (sometimes stresses which are difficult for the examiner to define), resulting in psychotic symptoms.

iii. Once treated acutely, usually with antipsychotic medication and/or specialized psychotherapy (see *Medication* and *Psychotherapies* sections), the patient can return to his former environment, with some continuing capacity for nonpsychotic adaptation within it.

iv. Adequate follow-up is important.

c. Psychotic episodes which are brief or extended portions of an ongoing conflict with reality (chronic psychosis) in which the acute episode is a *worsening rather than a change* of reality orientation:

i. These include schizophrenia, severe affective psychosis (e.g., manic-depressive disorder), and paranoid state disorders.

ii. Chronic medical intervention, usually medication, is often necessary to maintain a subacute status quo.

II.E: MENTAL RETARDATION

Severe retardation due to congenital and/or genetic factors is relatively easy to spot and the nonpsychiatric physician is rarely called upon for definitive treatment. One should be alert, however, for the patient who is "retarded" because of social deprivation or communication difficulty (dyslexias, deafness). Such a patient, if suspected in time and referred for special testing, can show significant gains, sometimes to full capacity, after appropriate intervention.

Retardation or lack of intellectual sophistication may lead to more than the usual apprehension or agitation in medical settings. Much of this can be avoided and the patient made more comfortable by the previously mentioned nonthreatening approaches (careful explanation, soft voice, etc.), sometimes much as one might approach a child.

Remember, however, that the retarded individual has feelings of competence and self-worth just as do other patients. He should be allowed to participate in his treatment, sit in on conferences about his condition, etc. Conversations in his presence should be *with* him rather than "about" him, a recommendation which applies to other patients as well.

Treatment in cases of moderate to severe retardation may occasionally call for institutional placement, but many services are often available within the local community. In any event, programs should be individualized and offer the best available opportunity for:

1. treatment of underlying medical disorders;
2. treatment of overlying emotional and adjustment problems;
3. the "pursuit of happiness" which is the patient's right; and
4. realization of maximum social, educational, and vocational potentials.

II.F: ALCOHOL ABUSE

1. Acute Intoxication

The inebriated person should not be referred for psychiatric consultation—whether to discuss withdrawal or treatment for alcoholism, to rule out other mental disease, or to cover the ER physician who feels he needs a consult before discharging the patient. There may be medical reason to observe the individual—to rule out other sources of intoxicated-appearing behavior, to calm his agitation, etc.—but *it is not possible to complete even a marginally accurate mental status examination while the patient is acutely intoxicated.* Therefore:

a. Do not attempt to assess suicide potential.
b. Do not attempt to estimate depression or emotional overlay (except as may be possible from reliable history from other persons).
c. Do not accept statements of wanting to withdraw from alcohol or enter treatment programs (although referral to a detoxification center may be appropriate).
d. Do not admit to the hospital on a psychiatric or purely alcohol abuse basis without clear and reliable historical justification.

Evaluate alcohol abusers when they are sober.

2. Chronic Abuse Patterns

Many alcohol abuse patterns are recognized as different from or short of physical addiction. The hallmark of these non-addiction states is that they interfere, to a greater or lesser extent, with the productive life of the patient or with the well-being of those around him/her.

Treatment at this stage involves:

a. a patient who recognizes the problem and is strongly motivated to deal with it;
b. primarily psychotherapeutic intervention, often at points of social, interpersonal, financial or vocational importance (e.g., "company programs" that address alcohol abuse), and
c. frequent group or peer-group emphasis.

3. Addiction

Addiction to alcohol may not be immediately visible within the patient's personal life:

a. Alcohol intake sufficient to avoid withdrawal symptoms may be such a part of daily activity that work and social appearance is near normal to the casual observer.
b. When patients are brought to the hospital seriously injured or unconscious, the history should be carefully

explored for possible alcohol addiction since withdrawal symptoms a few hours after admission may create an unpleasant surprise for both patient and staff.

Remember the obvious: Do not slight questions about alcohol abuse in the medical history.

4. Withdrawal

Withdrawal reactions can manifest themselves in many ways:

a. Symptoms and signs vary considerably with respect to severity and timing. Increased severity may be expected in patients who:
   i. have adjusted to high blood alcohol concentrations;
   ii. have a history of severe abstinence symptoms;
   iii. are in poor physical or emotional health; or
   iv. are over 30 years of age.
b. Symptoms/signs are specifically related to lack of alcohol, not to any dietary or vitamin deficiency (which may, of course, also be present).
c. Symptoms/signs may be delayed, or may seem to appear *de novo,* if the patient has a covert source of alcohol which suddenly is cut off.
d. *Tremulousness and general CNS irritability* are the first signs, usually appearing within a few hours of the last alcohol intake. Other early symptoms include GI disturbance, weakness, sleep disturbance, mild to moderately excessive sympathetic activity, fever, and impaired cognition.
e. *Hallucinations* may then appear:
   i. commonly visual, in contrast to the usually auditory hallucinations seen with functional psychosis;
   ii. usually accompanied by a clear sensorium.
f. *Seizures* may occur, even after several days:
   i. Most occur within the first 24–48 hours.
   ii. Withdrawal seizures are not preventable with so-called "prophylactic" phenytoin (Dilantin).
   iii. *Status epilepticus* is a concern.

g. If seizures occur, more neurological exam is indicated, since alcoholic patients may be more than usually prone to other causes of convulsive activity (traumatic hematoma, etc.). This is an especially important consideration if seizures occur after delirium has appeared.

h. *Delirium tremens* is a relatively uncommon but very serious endstage of withdrawal:

   i. The patient need not pass through a stage of seizures to reach DT's.

   ii. DT's generally occur three to four days after cessation of alcohol intake.

   iii. DT's can be differentiated from the possible hallucinations of earlier stages by severely *clouded sensorium* (delirium) and *acute illness* of the patient (autonomic crisis with tachycardia, sweating, mydriasis, etc.).

   iv. DT's is most often preventable.

i. *Alcoholic hallucinosis* involves primarily auditory, schizophreniform hallucinations after five to ten days of abstinence. Although properly treated with neuroleptic medication (see *Medication* section), this state is unrelated to schizophrenia and will clear, requiring no chronic medication. Older patients, mostly males, may develop a more chronic paranoia which, like the hallucinosis, usually responds to medication.

Treatment of alcohol withdrawal (our recommended regimen):

a. hydration (often IV) (may need sodium restriction), but do not overhydrate;

b. vitamin supplement (especially thiamine, 100–200 mg. stat, then 50 mg. p.o. daily); and

c. generous doses, IM stat and then orally, of an anxiolytic/ CNS depressant such as chlordiazepoxide or diazepam. These

   i. are excellent calmatives (but oversedation is unwise);

   ii. prevent seizures; and

   iii. make excellent sleeping medications, with good REM activity.

iv. Oxazepam is not available in IM/IV form but may be used orally later because of its apparently lower hepatotoxicity.
d. Careful observation for neurologic and other medical signs, as well as for medication reactions and for surreptitious availability of alcohol, is important.

It should be noted that other physicians have success with other regimens, some involving barbiturates, chloral hydrate and/or paraldehyde, in addition to the supportive and hydrating measures outlined. Sleep is important, and flurazepam or another non-REM-suppressing drug may be needed.

A word of caution is in order regarding the frequent use of chlorpromazine and other antipsychotic medications in alcohol withdrawal. We avoid them because:

a. They decrease the seizure threshold.
b. Any psychotic manifestations are due primarily to CNS toxicity and environmental stimulation, and as such are best prevented without such potent neuroleptics. An exception is the hallucinolytic effect of haloperidol 5 mg. q. 4 H for brief periods.
c. While sedation and reduced anxiety are target effects of the anxiolytics, the antipsychotics (or "major tranquilizers") have these only as side effects.
d. Potent and long-lasting CNS depressant effects of antipsychotic meds may mask other important signs.

5. Chronic Alcohol Treatment Programs

Once your patient is sober, he or she may decide to pursue serious treatment. It behooves you to know how to put him or her in contact with the appropriate people or facility. Do not let a potentially treatable alcoholic "fall into the cracks" between the detoxification ward and the definitive treatment program.

a. If there is an alcoholic treatment program (not just detox) near you, learn about it and keep the telephone number handy.

b. Find out which psychiatrists and psychotherapists in your area specialize in the treatment of alcoholics and their families, so that the person to whom you refer the patient is not so likely to be one who will overtly or covertly reject him.

c. There is an Alcoholics Anonymous (and likely an Al Anon and AlaTeen) chapter nearby:

i. Remember that these folks have the best overall track record in the business.

ii. Those patients who refuse AA (or other programs) on "philosophical" grounds are usually really saying, "I'll get help if it's painless, quick, magic, and if I can fall back on my drinking if I need to."

Patients who say they want help and then refuse comprehensive, perhaps residential programs, may not be ready for serious help.

II.G: OTHER DRUG ABUSE

1. Acute Intoxication

This is similar to alcohol in that the mood or sensorium is altered to some extent, with greater or lesser impairment of CNS and other body functions. Specifics are discussed elsewhere. See *Emergencies* (pp. 16–17) and *Alcohol Abuse* (pp. 29–30) sections.

2. Chronic Abuse Patterns

Most chronic abuse patterns, including physical addictions, have in common a strong thread of self-destruction. Although stimulation, relief from pain, self-treatment of emotional disease, and the like are often cited as significant components of abuse patterns, the bottom line is most often injury to the self and/or to those around the abuser.

Table 1 illustrates gross ordinal relationships among some drug groups with respect to several ways of conceptualizing "destructive potential."

Drugs with the most, or most rapid, likelihood for physical damage may not be those often associated with the "drug culture." Two factors seem most important in determining inherent dangerousness:

a. *Medical toxicity,* with some attention to route of administration, and
b. ability of the user to form *tolerance,* at which point he or she requires increased doses in order to achieve desired effects.

Heroin, for example, is highly toxic and is usually taken via a dangerous route (IV); however, many users reach a point after which they need not continue to increase their dosage, allowing some retention of functioning. This characteristic is shared with meperidine and other opiates and synthetic opiates, with a larger percentage of users being able to avoid escalation beyond levels of non-function as the potency recedes from that of heroin. On the other hand, some compounds, such as some aromatic hydrocarbons (gasoline, paint thinner, some glues), are so toxic that relatively infrequent or temporary abuse can result in serious damage to one or more organ systems.

Finally, abuse of legally prescribed and over-the-counter drugs must be considered significant. Look for depression or other emotional problems in patients who depend upon even minor calmatives or sleep aids.

Treatment. Treatment of depression along with the drug-abuse target symptoms is often useful; an *understanding* of the ubiquitous depressive component is almost imperative for lasting success (see page 20).

3. Addiction and Withdrawal

The questions of physiological *vs.* psychological dependence *vs.* other abuse patterns are too complex to fully address here. Physical dependence may be more complex to treat and involve more medical intervention; however, the pattern of

TABLE 1: Gross Destructive Potential of Some Substances of Abuse*

1 = little, minor; 2 = some, moderate; 3 = much, serious; 4 = extreme

Substance	Personal Impact Potential			Overall Negative Societal Impact	
	Medical	Psychological	Physical Addiction	Jobs, Lost Days, Economy	Serious Crime
Alcohol	3	3	3	4	3
Amphetamines	2–3	2–3	2	2	2–3
Aromatic Hydrocarbons (paint thinner, gasoline, some glues)	4	3	1	1	1
Barbiturates	2–3	2	3	2	1
Benzodiazepines (diazepam, etc.)	1–2	2	1–2	1	1–2
Caffeine	1–2	1–2	1–2	1	1
Cocaine	2	2	2	1–2	1–2
Codeine	1–2	2	2–3	1	1–2
Hallucinogens (Pure LSD)	1	4	1	1	1
Hallucinogens (Street—including LSD, STP, PCP (see below), Peyote, Mescaline, etc., often mixed or "cut" with contaminants)	2–3	4	1	1–2	1–2
Hashish	1–2	2–3	2	1–2	2

Heroin (relatively uncontaminated street use)	3	4	3	4
Marijuana (cannibis)	1–2	1	1–2	1–2
Meprobamate	1–2	3	1	1
Methadone	1–2	4	1–2	2
Methaqualones	2	2–3	1–2	1
Morphine	2–3	3–4	1–2	2
OTC Sleeping Medications, etc.	1–2	1–2	1–2	1
PCP ("Angel Dust," etc.)	3	1	2–3	2–3
Synthetic Narcotics	2–3	3	1–2	2
Tobacco (inhaled)	3	2–3	3	1–2

* The author is aware of the varying definitions which exist for such terms as "destructive," "potential," "serious," "psychological," and "addiction." There are also differences of opinion regarding overall drug effects.

abuse and the self-destructive reasons that almost always accompany it are of primary importance in understanding addiction of any type. Withdrawal then becomes a sociomedical process with particular characteristics being associated with some substance groups.

Heroin and other opioids

Overdose is common for a variety of reasons (accidents within the family of a methadone user; unexpected purity of street heroin). Respiratory depression and other effects secondary to heroin, methadone, or other opioid overdose are rapidly reversed by 0.4. mg. naloxone IV which may be repeated in a few minutes if ineffective. Other sources of coma must be explored concomitantly, such as the easily-treatable hypoglycemic shock. Hints of opioid abuse may be:
a. history;
b. needle tracks (although there are other routes for administration); and
c. evidence of street remedies such as milk (in the mouth, or inflamed areas where it has been injected).

Withdrawal is uncomfortable but not usually a medical emergency. Typical of heroin or morphine are the following:

a. Sweating, lacrimation, sniffing, yawning, "shakes," and mydriasis occur within 8–12 hours of last dose.
b. Insomnia, GI symptoms, muscle spasm and the like begin 1–2 days after the last dose, peaking at about three days.
c. The syndrome subsides over 7–10 days.
d. Symptoms are similar with methadone but begin after 1–2 days and last up to several weeks.
e. Withdrawal syndromes in newborns of mothers addicted to heroin or methadone begin within 48 hours of birth and include tremors, irritability, vomiting, hypertonicity, and fever. More severe syndromes may include respiratory problems and/or convulsions.

Treatment can be done on an outpatient basis so long as there is no complicating issue such as:

    i. multiple drug abuse, especially involving sedatives or meprobamate;

    ii. pregnancy;

    iii. serious infection, or other serious illness (e.g., hepatic damage), or unless there is an ongoing, long-term residential treatment plan attached to the detoxification process.

a. Inpatient treatment is thus usually not indicated, since

    i. opioid withdrawal *per se* carries little risk of serious medical complications;

    ii. there is little or no difference in rates of lasting rehabilitation between patients detoxed in and out of the hospital; and

    iii. outpatient withdrawal is a generally simple and straightforward process.

b. Withdrawal using methadone as a substitute for other opioids:

    i. Estimates of level of addiction are not necessary.

    ii. Start with 10–20 mg. orally and watch for somnolence as a sign of too much methadone. May increase in increments up to maximum 20 mg. per 12-hour period for suppression of withdrawal symptoms.

    iii. After the first day, methadone may be taken q.d. or b.i.d.

    iv. Once stabilized, begin methadone withdrawal by decreasing dose 5 mg. per day or 20% (maximum) per day. Mild withdrawal symptoms may be seen.

    v. Treatment of methadone addiction (even if secondary to methadone maintenance) is similar but more gradual.

c. Withdrawal without methadone:

    i. May be carried out with benzodiazepine anxiolytics in fairly high doses (diazepam, chlordiazepoxide), for discomfort, sedation, and sleeplessness. Some centers routinely use chloral hydrate or other symptomatic meds.

ii. Chlorpromazine or other neuroleptics are of less use than anxiolytics and may introduce problems discussed elsewhere in the text.

iii. Potential for abuse of benzodiazepine prescriptions exists and should be considered; however, it is the author's opinion that small but adequate supplies of anxiolytics often represent the best compromise among the issues of safety, efficacy and abuse potential.

d. Withdrawal of infants requires more specialized information, available elsewhere. Addicted newborns require neonatological consultation.

Barbiturates, Methaqualone, other Sedative Hypnotics, Meprobamate

CNS hypersensitivity accompanying abrupt withdrawal from these drugs produces a serious risk of seizures and *status epilepticus,* even though the daily intake may in some cases have been only slightly above that of routine prescriptions (e.g., with meprobamate). Patients presenting for withdrawal or wishing assistance in getting off the drug(s) must be counseled to come into the hospital for careful titration and monitoring.

Diazepam, and to some extent the other benzodiazepines, are now known to have a withdrawal syndrome similar to, but not as severe as, the sedative-hypnotics, including occasional presence of seizures or, rarely, sudden respiratory arrest, even after several days. These syndromes apparently develop only with dosages above routine levels and can be averted by titrated detoxification. There seems reason to advocate hospitalization as a general rule for this high-dosage group.

If a patient is addicted to both an opioid and a sedative-hypnotic, maintain the opioid addiction while following the steps below to withdraw the sedative.

Treatment is as follows:

a. Determine the level of addiction via the *barbiturate tolerance test:*
   i. The barbiturates are cross-tolerant with all of the sedative-hypnotics and meprobamate and can thus be used for both accurate diagnosis and controlled withdrawal.
   ii. To an alert patient, give 200 mg. oral pentobarbital.
   iii. Examine after one hour for signs and symptoms listed in Table 2.
   iv. If no response, wait several hours and repeat with 300 mg. pentobarbital.
b. Withdraw with decreasing daily doses of pentobarbital:
   i. Phenobarbital may be substituted for pentobarbital at ⅓ the pentobarbital dose (see Table 2).

TABLE 2: Responses and Recommendations Following 200 mg. Oral Pentobarbital (Barbiturate Tolerance Test)

Exam After One Hour Shows:	Approximate Daily Dosage Requirement of:	
	Pentobarbital	Phenobarbital
Asleep (arousable)	none	none
Drowsy, slurred speech, ataxia, marked nystagmus, obviously intoxicated	400–600 mg.	120–200 mg.
Not obviously intoxicated but subtle neurological signs such as fine nystagmus	800–900 mg.	250–300 mg.
Alert, no overt or neurologic signs of intoxication; may even still have signs of withdrawal	1000 mg. or more	350 mg. or more
Alert as immediately above after 300 mg. test dose	1500 mg. or more	500 mg. or more

    ii. Divide daily doses into q.i.d. for pentobarbital, t.i.d. for phenobarbital.

    iii. Reduce at 10% per day.

    iv. Watch for CNS hyperirritability (indicating too rapid decrease) or somnolence (too much medication or surreptitious drug availability).

    v. Expect other withdrawal discomforts, including insomnia and REM rebound (often producing nightmares), sometimes for weeks.

  c. In emergencies of impending withdrawal, give 100–200 mg. IM phenobarbital, then begin oral tests and treatment several hours after any toxic signs abate.

4. Ongoing Treatment Programs

Some programs are quite anti-chemical and many are criticized (as is AA) for replacing chemical dependency with dependency upon a program or set of beliefs.

  a. The physician should be prepared to follow up acute detoxification with appropriate referral for ongoing, perhaps residential treatment.

  b. The physician should be aware of the *methods* and *efficacy* of the various drug rehabilitation programs in his or her area, since the field is replete with people "doing their own thing," often ex-addicts who for one reason or another find themselves in the thick of solving the problems of human suffering and are often able to get others to finance or support them.

  c. The referring physician should be able to satisfy himself that the end result is likely to be patient benefit, whatever the orientation of program or treatment.

  d. After detoxification, be alert for the same kinds of excuses and rationalizations as those seen in the alcoholic, although these may take different forms reflecting the varying social characteristics of the patient populations.

II.H: SEXUAL PROBLEMS

Sexual problems may be embarrassing for the patient, and unfortunately sometimes for the physician, to discuss. They can
be frightening for the patient, especially for the male patient
who may feel that his masculinity is threatened. At various
times, sexual problems can be either *disruptive to* family relationships or *precipitated by* couple or family difficulties. Sexual
dysfunction may be part of an unconscious *adaptation* to a
particular relationship, and thus be difficult for the patient to
give up. Often the patient wishes it were a medical problem or
the other partner's fault. Sometimes it is. Occasionally, a
condition defined by the patient as a "problem" may not be seen
as such by the physician. This may occur when the patient is
concerned about something which the physician, after a careful history, often involving both partners, considers "normal."
Such situations should be handled with explanation and/or
exploration to the patient's satisfaction (not the doctor's). The
need for information regarding sex may be the most common
sexual concern seen in the usual general practice.

1. Premature Ejaculation

This dysfunction is:

   a. Very common, although often unreported.
   b. "Premature" generally means an inability to postpone
      ejaculation long enough to:
      i. enter the vagina,
      ii. sustain further arousal of the woman, and
      iii. thrust forcefully and long enough to result in mutual
          pleasure in a majority of episodes of coitus.

Treatment:

   a. Many psychodynamic explanations may be present and
      may be therapeutically explored; however,
   b. substantial improvement in a majority of cases is pos-
      sible by means of the "squeeze technique" first described
      by James Semans at the University of Virginia. This is a

simple technique taught via drawings or photos to both sexual partners. Although easy to employ, the technique should be taught by qualified persons who have a working knowledge of the principles involved and who are skilled in couples therapy.

2. Male Erectile Impotence

a. Impotence is common, but less specific in its presentation or treatment than is premature ejaculation.
b. Impotence may be defined as an inability to achieve or maintain an erection of sufficient firmness and duration for satisfactory coitus. The condition may be further defined as primary—i.e., long-standing and without apparent physical cause—or secondary.
c. Presentation may involve:
   i. lack of arousal,
   ii. lack of erectile ability, or
   iii. loss of erection before or soon after entry.
d. Physical factors should be explored, and may involve medical illness (including alcohol abuse), trauma, or iatrogenic causes (e.g., medications).
e. Most cases are due to emotional factors such as:
   i. worry about one's sexual performance or the partner's expectations,
   ii. unconscious anger with the partner or someone she represents,
   iii. subtle preoccupation with one's life stresses (e.g., work), or
   iv. clinical or masked *depression*.
f. A key question in the history may be whether or not the male can *ever* achieve erection.

Treatment may be facilitated by:

a. sex education and reassurance (see below);
b. supportive counseling;
c. brief environmental change; or

d. low doses of anxiolytic medication.

e. Since impotence may be a symptom of depression or emotional conflict, psychotherapeutic and pharmacologic treatments for underlying causes (see elsewhere in text) should be considered.

f. Although many cases of impotence, especially "primary" impotence, seem difficult to treat, those who do not respond to the above within a reasonable time may be referred to a reputable treatment center with some optimism.

As with other psychosomatic difficulties, telling the patient that it's "all in his head" or that he "shouldn't try so hard" is worthless. Support and a sharing of the understanding that virtually all men have temporary impotence at some point in their lives may be of considerable help.

3. Females with Insufficient Orgasm

a. The term "frigid" is inappropriate and obsolete. Truly anorgasmic females are rare; lack of orgasm may not be related to the woman's capacity for sexual response.

b. It is inappropriate to view female arousal or orgasm as any less "important" than that of the male. Education—perhaps including education of the partner—may be very helpful, provided it is undertaken by a knowledgeable, non-threatening physician or therapist.

c. Careful history is needed to determine:
   i. whether the patient has ever experienced orgasm,
   ll. whether she knows what an orgasm is or feels like for her,
   iii. whether systemic illness is present (e.g., diabetes),
   iv. whether coitus is painful, and
   v. whether birth control is an issue or worry.

Treatment: A few medical causes of dyspareunia and lack of orgasm are publicized (hooded clitoris, occluded introitus, endometriosis, etc.), perhaps as part of the need for "magical" answers to uncomfortable questions. Most women are free of these and can learn to experience orgasm. Some do well with specialized orgasm training groups which may stress specific masturbation techniques, Kegel's exercises, sharing of feelings among women with similar concerns, and couples-oriented counseling. Again, it behooves the physician to know of *reputable* referral professionals in his community.

4. Stereotypes and Myths

Adult sexual activity is generally considered "normal" so long as it:

a. satisfies one's perceived needs;
b. avoids purposeful pain or injury to, or intrusion upon others; and
c. is carried out with adults. Conditions which fill these three criteria and are not presented to the physician by the patient as a "problem" should not be treated as pathological or discouraged unless they are felt to be medically contraindicated.

Children and adolescents should be supportively guided and assisted—with ample opportunity for privacy—in their exploration of their sexuality, since this is a confusing and sometimes frightening set of experiences. Sexual feelings, activities and experimentation among age-appropriate peers are generally normal; however, adult-child or adolescent-child activities are likely indications of emotional disturbance, usually in the older person, and may be harmful to the child.

"Normality" is sometimes an issue when considering the *elderly* or the *disabled*. There should be no doubt that these two groups have as much right—and often as much ability—to enjoy sex as does the rest of the population. Concepts that can allow the physician to understand, discuss, and assist with the sexual concerns of his patients include awareness that:

a. Erectile and orgasmic ability usually extend into senescence.

b. One need not use a penis and/or vagina in order to bring pleasure to a partner.

c. Even the neurologically flaccid penis may be capable of stimulation and ejaculation.

d. Erectile ability and a number of other physical characteristics often have little to do with one's ability to father or conceive children.

e. The world is full of satisfying approaches to sexual fulfillment so long as one is free to consider them. With such understanding, the physician will be able to frankly and realistically approach with the patient potential alterations in or loss of sexual function which may accompany aging, illness, or trauma.

5. Perversions and Aberrations

a. As above, any sexual problem, even if considered "normal" by the physician, is a problem for the patient if it presents as such.

b. Such complaints may be used by the patient as an *entrée* into counseling, a starting point for talking about problems in seemingly unrelated areas.

c. Often the problem will be presented to the family physician by a concerned spouse.

   i. If the problem does not involve injury to others, the physician should voice his availability to help but wait for the identified patient to seek treatment.

   ii. If some sort of injury is suspected or occurring (e.g., child or wife abuse), the physician should meet with the couple in order to bring the problem out into the open and increase motivation for treatment.

d. Although the physician should offer to listen to and talk about sexual problems with the patient, and should be able to offer referral for more detailed counseling, one should be alert for the patient who is looking for a magical cure which can never be found. The physician should never promise such a cure.

6. Legal Aspects

Forensic presentations of sexual aberrations are not uncommon. Often the police or family will bring an offender for evaluation just after he is apprehended. In other cases the individual may come to the family doctor or emergency room psychiatric section on the advice of his attorney. Such requests for evaluation or treatment should be approached with some caution, even though you may be pressed for premature professional opinions.

It is useful to separate offenses into those which are violent (forcible rape, physical assault) and those which are not (exhibitionism, voyeurism, etc.). Perpetrators of the latter acts:

a. Are rarely an immediate danger to anyone.
b. Their disorders may be chronic and difficult to treat.
c. Handling of the acute situation is usually best accomplished by calming everyone down pending further workup and settlement of legal matters, although one should not attempt to minimize the concerns expressed or add to the patient's need to deny the problem.
d. These patients should not be admitted to the hospital *unless you feel they are so embarrassed or depressed that there is a risk of suicide attempt.*

Violent offenders:

a. Should be initially handled within the legal system, since they may represent a danger to others, and
b. Should not be hospitalized unless suicidal.
c. If inpatient evaluation is needed, it should be done via court order.

Other factors that are useful in early evaluation and disposition have to do with whether children are involved as victims, whether incest is an issue, and whether alcohol or other drugs seem part of the alleged offense.

In the case of pedophilic offenses, including incest, the anger of the involved adults (parents, police officers) may cloud salient issues. The offenders are usually docile, ineffectual people who should be handled with professional care within the confines of their legal situation.

In incest, the identified offender may be a scapegoat for a morass of family problems, leading to a need for the family to place all its troubles and blame on the offender and/or the victim. Detailed family evaluation is necessary.

Involvement of alcohol (or other drugs) in sexual crimes is a complex but very important issue. The alcohol may be an excuse to free the inner self from its conscience, a sign of serious depression, or part of a chemically-mediated organic dyscontrol syndrome. A complete history and evaluation are necessary in order to unravel its role in the offense.

7. Victims of Sexual Crimes

    a. Victims deserve immediate, competent attention.

    b. The victim has suffered what is, at best, an unwarranted intrusion and, at worst, sudden physical injury.

    c. The physician should be considerate of the victim and try to minimize the trauma and its sequelae, even though a thorough examination and workup may be necessary.

    d. This is especially important in the case of children, even though the concept of one's being "scarred for life" by a single sexual trauma is often overrated:

        i. The event should be discussed with the child.

        ii. All attendant feelings should be allowed to come out over time.

        iii. The child must be supported in his/her attempts to regain lost self-image, conquer fears, overcome guilts, etc.

        iv. Families must not foster a concept of "dirtiness" in the child.

        v. The child should never be asked or required to "keep quiet" for the family's sake, as is often the case in incest.

Never underestimate the destructive power of the "family secret" or of subtle punitiveness that a family may lay upon the shoulders of the child.

Finally, it is not uncommon for a person to present to the physician with a sexual confession of sorts, usually of a minor perversion. You should listen with compassion but with some caution, since this may be a patient who is about to be arrested or tried and he may be using you for legal weight rather than for any real help.

The crux of these comments regarding forensic presentations is that one must take the time to unravel as many facts as possible, if appropriate to do so at the time of presentation. Talk with everyone involved, including children, and don't forget the victim. It is most often the case that the acute presentation is not the place for any long evaluation or definitive decisions.

III Psychotropic Medications

III.A: ANTIPSYCHOTIC DRUGS

NOTE: Recommendations in this section are meant for *adults*. Psychotropic medication of children should generally be done only by a specialist (see *Children,* Chapter VIII:B).

There are two main groups: *neuroleptics* for acute and chronic functional psychosis (and selected organic psychoses), and *lithium,* which is generally limited to use in severe affective disorders, especially mania. Antidepressants also have antipsychotic properties but are discussed separately (III.B).

1. Neuroleptics

These drugs are all similar in that they are

    a. active within the CNS, probably at the neurotransmitter level, to reduce symptoms of psychosis;
    b. central adrenergic blockers;
    c. metabolized in the liver and hence potentially hepatotoxic; and
    d. CNS depressants.

Chemical classes include

    a. phenothiazines—many forms, widest popularity;
    b. butyrophenones—haloperidol (Haldol) in U.S.A.;
    c. thioxanthenes—fairly new, similar to above in concept;
    d. dihydroindolones and dibenzoxazepines—both quite new and purported to offer fewer (or different) side effects than other neuroleptics. Therapeutic efficacy, long-term

clinical experience, and/or reasons to choose these above the more experienced compounds are yet to be completely established.

Table 3 highlights some important characteristics of representative examples of these and other psychoactive drug classes. Recently introduced compounds are treated somewhat vaguely, both in the table and in the text.

The following are generally useful treatment regimens for three situations involving functional, schizophrenic-like psychotic illness.

Treatment of acute psychosis in which the patient is *known to have an exacerbation of a functional psychotic disorder* may be undertaken with either of the *"rapid tranquilization formulas"* below.

a. Haloperidol (Haldol)
   i. Start with 5 mg. IM (or 10 mg. orally).
   ii. Observe for *hypotension* and sedation.
   iii. Repeat hourly or q2h in 10 mg. increments with close observation, until symptoms subside or sedation occurs.
   iv. Do not exceed 60 mg. in 12 hours or 100 mg. in 24 hours.
   v. Continuing this acute regimen beyond 12 hours is not recommended without careful consideration of relative benefits and potential dangers.
   vi. Haloperidol probably carries less danger of hypotensive complications and shows earlier antipsychotic effects than does chlorpromazine (below). It is less sedating and may in high doses exceed a "threshold," lowering the incidence and severity of extrapyramidal (basal ganglionic) side effects.
b. Chlorpromazine (Thorazine, etc.)
   i. 50 mg. IM.
   ii. Observe closely for 30 minutes for hypotension and sedation.
   iii. Repeat if necessary and medically safe (may use 100 mg. IM if manic).

   iv. Observe for one hour.

   v. Repeat hourly until calming occurs or side effects preclude further dosage.

   vi. Do not exceed 300 mg. IM without clear documentation of need and safety.

The above may allow ER treatment of acute psychosis which would formerly have required days or weeks of hospitalization; however, follow-up maintenance medication and contact are necessary (see below). A more *conservative alternative* for acute treatment might include:

a. observation without meds for several hours (especially if drug intoxication is suspected); then

b. oral antipsychotic med in moderate doses, e.g., 400 mg. chlorpromazine daily, divided b.i.d. or t.i.d.

   i. The above avoids the physical and emotional side effects of IM route.

   ii. Watch for side effects and add antiparkinsonian meds PRN.

   iii. Use meds with sedative side effects if needed.

   iv. Use only one antipsychotic at a time; combinations are rarely indicated.

c. Increase med every day or two as needed, up to maximum dose (1000+ mg. oral chlorpromazine or equivalent per day). The sedative effect starts early; however, antipsychotic effect may be delayed up to two or three weeks.

d. If desired remission does not occur, consider switching to another med, perhaps of a different chemical group (little or no "washout" time is needed with antipsychotics).

e. Once remission has begun, consider decreasing dosage to subacute levels outlined below.

NOTE: Epinephrine should be avoided in the treatment of neuroleptic-induced hypotension. Levarterenol or phenylephrine may be used but is rarely needed. In case of cardiac arrest in a patient coincidentally taking neuroleptics, epinephrine is recommended.

Management of semi-acute functional psychosis of a non-affective type (most frequently schizophrenia or related diagnosis) during the recompensation stages can sometimes be done on an outpatient basis but often requires two to four weeks of hospitalization.

a. Treatment should include *one* of the above meds (or a related one) in addition to a therapeutic milieu (see *Psychotherapies* section).

b. Side effects and route of administration may be factors in choosing meds (see Tables 3 and 5).
   i. Oral routes tend to be best if feasible.
   ii. Surreptitious medications (e.g., in the patient's food) or forcing of meds in an assaultive way should be avoided.
   iii. Sedative side effects are undesirable after the first few days.

c. Extrapyramidal side effects may be approached via antiparkinsonian drugs in two ways:
   i. prophylactically, which may prevent problems and enhance patient compliance *but* will be medicating a number of patients who wouldn't have needed it and possibly decreasing effectiveness of antipsychotic meds; or
   ii. symptomatically, which treats only those patients who need the antiparkinsonian med *but* allows uncomfortable and/or disquieting side effects to develop in a group of patients who may therefore later be reluctant to take needed antipsychotic meds.
   iii. In any event, the antiparkinsonians can and should be reduced or eliminated after tolerance has developed to the antipsychotic medication.

d. Underdosage, in terms both of amount and duration of medication, is common among nonpsychiatric physicians in acute-care hospitals. Levels recommended in the **PDR** tend to be quite conservative for schizophreniform psychoses.

e. Once-daily doses are almost always appropriate once

initial symptoms have abated. Such dosage schedules

  i. are more convenient for everyone concerned;
 ii. encourage better patient compliance, especially after discharge; and
iii. give fewer reminders of patient's "sick" or "dependent" status.
 iv. Except as noted in Table 3, all antipsychotics (and tricyclic antidepressants and many antiparkinsonians) have sufficiently long half-lives to allow q.d. dosage without resorting to the more expensive "sequels," "P.M.," "spansule" or other advertised "timed release" forms.

f. IM depot medication (fluphenazine enanthate or decanoate) may be useful and convenient; however, it is not without emotional effects (e.g., taking control of treatment away from the patient) and has a very high incidence of anticholinergic and extrapyramidal symptoms. The antipsychotic effect lasts about two weeks with the enanthate form, slightly longer with the decanoate, *as do any side effects* that accompany the drug. It is often wise to test fluphenazine tolerance orally for a few days before using the depot preparation.

Chronic Treatment of Functional Schizophreniform Psychoses. Goals should be to maximize length of remissions, improve quality of life, and avoid serious adverse effects of long-term neuroleptic medication. The typical patient is often one who:

a. has been hospitalized more than once;
b. may require further hospitalization every few months or years;
c. has settled into an existence in semi-institutional surroundings (board and care home, rooming house) or become a less-than-productive part of a family setting (although this is not always the case and good treatment can often result in a productive future); and
d. is *infantilized* by his surroundings and his disability.

Medication:

a. is central to good treatment and prevention of symptom relapse;
b. should be combined with good nutrition and proper attendance to the social and environmental needs of the patient;
c. should usually be continued indefinitely or discontinued only with careful monitoring of the patient with the understanding that psychotic symptoms will likely reappear;
d. should be maintained at the lowest effective dose, adjusted lower as the patient becomes elderly;
e. may be varied among different chemical groups from time to time;
f. may be temporarily discontinued for a few days at a time (drug holidays).

Tardive dyskinesia is a progressive, often non-reversible neuromuscular syndrome which can appear as a reaction to chronic neuroleptic medication. The syndrome resembles levodopa toxicity and some rare neuromuscular problems of senescence. Iatrogenic tardive dyskinesia is probably due to basal ganglionic rebound phenomena secondary to prolonged dopaminergic (or other adrenergic) blockade. The physician hopes to minimize or prevent it by means of the last three *caveats* (d., e., f.) listed above.

Early symptoms of tardive dyskinesia may appear in any patient taking neuroleptic medication, but are more common in elderly, chronically medicated patients. Initially one may see:

a. perioral movements, mouthings, tongue thrusting;
b. blinking, facial grimacing;
c. vermicular movement of the tongue.

These may progress to neck and truncal dyskinesias, or to choreoathetoid movements of the extremities. Symptoms will increase with emotional tension or stress, and will virtually always disappear when the patient is sleeping.

Symptoms of tardive dyskinesia increase with tension and disappear when the patient is asleep.

Treatment:

a. Tardive dyskinesia is usually not reversible, although some remission may take place after several weeks or months without neuroleptic medication.
b. Antiparkinsonian drugs are of no lasting benefit and may make things worse.
c. A decision must be made with respect to the patient's need for neuroleptic medication *vs* the slow progression of the dyskinesia:
    i. Decreased dose or change of chemical group may slow or stop the progression.
    ii. Stopping neuroleptic meds will arrest the progress of the dyskinesia, *even though symptoms may become temporarily worse immediately after discontinuance.*
    iii. Increasing the neuroleptic medication will seem to make symptoms better, since the adrenergic "rebound" will be stifled; however, *this will only set the stage for worse symptoms in the long run.*
    iv. A number of medical treatments are being studied at this time; however, none is well established or FDA approved.
d. Prevention and periodic examination for early symptoms remain the best approaches for minimizing disability.
    i. Use the lowest effective dose of medication.
    ii. Try to avoid the use of antiparkinsonian preparations in chronic patients.
    iii. Keep in mind the fact that many authorities feel that the development of tardive dyskinesia is correlated with total dose of neuroleptic medication over time.

Other long-term considerations for chronic neuroleptic treatment include weight gain and subtle changes in physical appearance, subtle CNS toxicity and chronic changes in a number of chemical and hormonal balances. Most of these are benign and/or of little significance given the seriousness of the diagnosis and the ability of the medication to decrease symptoms and increase quality of life. The dull appearance, dry hair, intellectual deterioration, etc., that were once thought to characterize the chronic schizophrenic need not be nearly so common with minimized effective dosages, better nutrition and better social/vocational opportunity.

2. Lithium Carbonate

This medication:

    a. is specific for certain *affective* disorders;
    b. treats and prevents *manic* phase of manic-depressive disorder;
    c. prevents depressive phase but does not effectively treat it;
    d. has some experimental uses in other disorders, e.g., aggressive ones; and
    e. is excreted via the kidneys rather than the liver.

In the *treatment* of manic and hypomanic phases:

    a. high doses of neuroleptics may be necessary for control of acute mania;
    b. lithium carbonate can rapidly be substituted when the diagnosis is established;
    c. baseline thyroid studies (TSH, T4, T3 resin uptake, free T4 index, serum thyroid antibodies), renal function tests (BUN, creatinine, 24-hour creatinine clearance if indicated) and EKG should precede lithium prescription (see Table 3).
    d. Initiation of treatment:
        i. Begin with 300 mg. t.i.d. in physically normal adults.
        ii. Serum Li^+ should be between 0.6 and 1.2 meq/1.
        iii. Therapeutic levels are very close to toxic levels. Toxic effects may begin at or below 1.3 meq/1 (GI upset, diarrhea, fine tremor, thirst, polyuria).
        iv. Initially, serum levels should be drawn daily, then q.o.d., until stable.

      v. Levels should be determined from serum drawn at least 6–8 hours after last dose (e.g., in morning before first dose).

  e. Maintenance:

      i. Serum levels should be taken every 4–6 weeks.

      ii. Levels can be altered by patient noncompliance, dietary changes, minor physical illness.

      iii. Once maintenance is established there are few patient complaints. There is no dulling of mood, persistent anticholinergic effect, etc., as often seen with the previously discussed neuroleptics.

      iv. TSH every 3 months for the first year will help predict hypothyroid problems, which occur—usually asymptomatically—in about 5% of patients on lithium.

  f. Early side effects and adverse reactions:

      i. One is dealing with a potentially psychotic patient and a non-benign drug; so the patient should not be given control of his meds prematurely.

      ii. Early temporary side effects are occasional (see Table 3).

      iii. Conditions which alter serum sodium levels or compromise hydration even for a day or two must be watched for by both physician and patient.

      iv. Cardiovascular and thyroid effects are summarized in Table 3.

III.B: ANTIDEPRESSANT DRUGS

Of the two main classes of antidepressants—not including stimulants, which are not primarily antidepressant—only one, the tricyclic group, is in common usage in this country. The other class, the monoamine oxidase inhibitors (MAOI), have useful properties but are rarely initial drugs of choice because of side effects, dietary considerations (imperative avoidance of high-tyramine foods), and incompatibility with many other drugs (see *Drug Interactions,* Table 5). Certain refractory depressions may be treated first with a tricycle antidepressant and then with an added MAO inhibitor. *This practice is not recommended for nonpsychiatric physicians.* This section will not address the use of MAOI's.

The dibenzazepine-derived antidepressants, commonly known as tricyclics, represent the bulk of antidepressants prescribed or recommended. They have a lot in common as a group, including dosage schedules, therapeutic action and side effects. They facilitate central adrenergic transmission and are strongly anticholinergic.

Patients most likely to respond favorably to tricyclics are:

a. Those in whom the depression is not primarily situational and is severe enough to justify the use of potent medication. This may include:
   i. depressive phases of manic-depressive disorders;
   ii. involutional depressions;
   iii. severe and lasting post-partum depressions;
   iv. other severe depressions as described in *Presentations* section.

b. Patients with the "vegetative signs" of depression described in the *Presentations* section, including:
   i. anorexia,
   ii. weight loss,
   iii. psychomotor retardation,
   iv. early morning awakening.

c. Patients with a family history of depression which has responded to a particular tricyclic.

Using these criteria, some 60–80% of patients will improve, provided:

a. *Dosage* is adequate (with good patient compliance):
   i. 75–225 mg./day maintenance for healthy adults for all tricyclics except,
   ii. Protriptyline (Vivactyl) 30–60 mg./day, and
   iii. Nortriptyline (Aventyl) 40–80 mg./day.
   iv. *Note: Plasma level* of active antidepressant is the primary criterion for adequate dosage. Since this level may vary greatly from patient to patient even when

TABLE 3: Common Characteristics of Representative Antipsychotic and Antidepressant Drugs

I. NEUROLEPTICS—Generic name is followed by common brand name in parentheses.

Drug	Common Side Effects	Serious Dangers (see also Emergencies)	Comments
Chlorpromazine—Aliphatic side chain (Thorazine)	Sedation, extrapyramidal symptoms (tremor, rigidity, akathisia, dysarthria), anticholinergic symptoms (dry mouth, blurred vision, etc.), heat intolerance, photosensitivity, orthostatic hypotension, occasional dystonias in younger patients. Occasional skin rash, pruritis.	Hypotension (especially IM—do not use epinephrine—see text), decreased seizure threshold, tardive dyskinesia with long-term use, additive effects with CNS depressants, (alcohol, anesthetics, sedatives, analgesics). Very rare agranulocytosis.	Acute oral dose = 200–1000 mg/day; (usually less for maintenance). IM dose = ½ oral dose or less. Hepatic metabolism (hepatotoxic), strongly antiemetic, as are other phenothiazines, and may mask GI symptoms (as may all antipsychotics and antidepressants except lithium).
Thioridazine—Piperidine side chain (Mellaril)	Similar to chlorpromazine but fewer extrapyramidal ("parkinsonian") symptoms. More complaints of prostate and libido problems.	As above, and serious danger of significant retinopathy in doses over 800 mg/day; probably more cardiotoxic.	Limited dosage range; may be useful when extrapyramidal side effects are an issue.
Trifluoperazine—Piperazine side chain (Stelazine)	Similar to chlorpromazine but little sedation; more extrapyramidal symptoms, especially akathisia.	Similar to chlorpromazine.	Nonsedating; blocks proportionally more dopamine than chlorpromazine.
Fluphenazine—Piperazine side chain (Prolixin)	Similar to chlorpromazine but little sedation. Much parkinsonism. More extrapyramidal side effects, especially akathisia.	Similar to chlorpromazine but probably more long-term danger of dyskinesia.	Nonsedating. Depot IM form available. Stronger dopamine blocker.

P H E N O T H I A Z I N E S

Drug	Common Side Effects	Serious Dangers (see also Emergencies)	Comments
Haloperidol (Haldol)—A butyrophenone	More extrapyramidal effects, less sedation. More reports of patient intolerance. Otherwise similar to piperazine side chain phenothiazines.	Similar to the piperazine phenothiazines. Perhaps less hepatotoxic and less danger of agranulocytosis.	Very potent. IM form especially useful in acute psychosis. Strong dopamine blocker. Drug of choice in Gilles de la Tourette syndrome.
Thiothixene (Navane)—A thioxanthene	Similar to chlorpromazine but less sedation.	Similar to chlorpromazine.	Perhaps better patient acceptance than phenothiazines. May be useful in cases responding poorly to phenothiazines or haloperidol.
Loxapine (Loxitane)—A dibenzoxazepine	Extrapyramidal and anticholinergic symptoms. Somewhat sedative.	Probably similar to phenothiazines.	Recently introduced. May need divided doses rather than once-daily as in all of the above. Probably best chosen as an alternative when the above are insufficient.
Molindone (Moban)—A dihydroindolone	May have fewer extrapyramidal symptoms, perhaps less decrease in seizure threshold. Somewhat sedative.	Long-term effects are not yet clear. Probably similar to phenothiazines.	Quite new. Probably less effectively antipsychotic than the above. Doesn't interfere with guanethidine (unlike all of the above). Calcium in the preparation may alter gut absorption of meds such as tetracycline and phenytoin. May require divided doses.

II. LITHIUM CARBONATE—(Eskalith, Lithane, Lithonate)	Possible initial GI upset, fine tremor, thirst, polyuria, lethargy, all generally transient. EKG and thyroid changes may occur but are usually benign.	Toxic dose is close to therapeutic dose. Electrolyte imbalance and concomitant arrhythmias common if patient is dehydrated, has lowered sodium intake, or has increased sodium excretion (e.g., with diuretics).	Serum level must be monitored and patient educated to danger signs (see text). Divided doses of 300 to 600 mg t.i.d. for a total of 900 to 1800 mg/day, in order to reach serum levels of 0.6 to 1.2 meq/l. Baseline EKG and thyroid studies recommended before use. Concomitant diuretic use is contraindicated.

III. ANTIDEPRESSANTS—tricyclics

Imipramine (Imavate, SK-Pramine, Tofranil)—tertiary amine	Anticholinergic and autonomic effects, especially in elderly, including orthostatic hypotension, constipation, occasional EKG changes, prostate problems.	Suicide from overdose (see text); cardiac, liver, and CNS toxicity (especially in the elderly).	Imipramine and amitriptyline may represent two subclasses of tricyclics which treat two physiologically separate kinds of depression. A patient who is a "nonresponder" to one (or others like it) may respond well to the other. Additive with CNS depressants. Neither is an "activator" as often advertised. As with all tricyclics, once-daily dosage is sufficient after first few days.
Amitriptyline (Elavil, Endep)—tertiary amine	Similar to imipramine but more sedative.	Similar to imipramine.	
Doxepin (Adapin, Sinequan)	Similar to imipramine but perhaps milder and is more sedative.	Similar to imipramine but less cardiotoxic.	Purported to treat mixed anxiety and depression. Fewer side effects but probably less real antidepressant activity.
Protriptyline (Vivactil)	Similar to imipramine.	Similar to imipramine.	Most potent tricyclic (2.5 times the above drugs), but still does not "activate" the patient.

identical oral dosages are given, the above dose ranges should be seen as approximate.

b. *Duration* of medication trial is sufficient (4 or more weeks).

c. Duration of medication maintenance *after improvement has plateaued* should be at least several months; then taper and watch for relapse.

Other considerations that further increase chances of therapeutic success include:

a. First trying drugs from the amitriptyline-like (tertiary amine) group if agitation is present; or

b. Starting with the imipramine-like (tertiary amine) group in "retarded" depression; or

c. Switching from one group to another if the first is unsuccessful after 3–4 weeks of trial.

d. In particularly severe or psychotic depression, some clinicians add a neuroleptic, usually thioridazine, in moderately low doses.

e. Liothyronine (Cytomel) has also been advocated as an

TABLE 4: Relative Antipsychotic Potency Compared to Chlorpromazine (Oral Administration)

Drug and (Common Trade Names)	Oral Dosage Approx. Equivalent to 100 mg. Chlorpromazine (mg.)
Thioridazine (Mellaril)	100 mg.
Mesoridazine (Serentil)	50
Trifluoperazine (Stelazine)	5+
Fluphenazine (Prolixin)	2+
Haloperidol (Haldol)	2+
Thiothixene (Navane)	5–10[1]
Chlorprothixene (Taractan)	50–75[1]
Loxapine (Loxitane)	10–20[2]
Molindone (Moban)	10–15[2]

1. Thioxanthene compounds; may not be directly comparable to chlorpromazine.

2. Newer compounds; estimates are vague and may not be comparable.

adjunct, especially in women, but its efficacy is questionable.

f. Addition of trifluoperazine (Stelazine) in low doses—if improvement is slow—is advocated by some. If this is done, we recommend that it be dispensed separately, rather than in a "fixed dose" preparation such as Triavil or Etrafon.

The tricyclics are among the most toxic and potentially dangerous of psychotropic drugs.

a. Toxic dose is fairly close to therapeutic dose, especially in the elderly.
b. Cardiovascular, hepatic, and CNS effects must be kept in mind (see Table 3).
c. In older patients consider:
   i. pre-drug EKG,
   ii. lowered starting and maintenance doses,
   iii. Doxepin, which is less cardiotoxic (but perhaps less antidepressant),
   iv. divided doses to minimize anticholinergic load.
d. To minimize side effects and their interference with treatment:
   i. Start with lower doses and increase over 1–3 weeks.
   ii. Educate patients to expect mild side effects and to expect most to subside within a few days or weeks.
   iii. Use once-daily doses, perhaps in evening, once maintenance levels are reached.
e. Drug interactions must be kept in mind (see Table 5), since patients in need of antidepressants are likely to have concomitant medical illness.

This group of patients are among the most likely to attempt suicide. Tricyclics can be lethal in even moderate overdose (1 gram or more—less with protriptyline and nortriptyline—depending upon the patient's physical condition and idiosyncratic factors). Be sure you know your patient well before giving a large supply of medication, and remember that

the early recovering depressed patient may be likely to mobilize previously inactive suicidal thoughts.

III.C: ANXIOLYTICS ("MINOR TRANQUILIZERS")

Although a number of medications are used for alleviation of anxiety, only three groups—meprobamate, hydroxyzine, and the benzodiazepines—are useful anxiolytics. Barbiturates, antihistamines, neuroleptics, and the host of other drugs, over-the-counter and prescription, that are sometimes used as anxiolytics should not be used in the treatment of uncomplicated anxiety.

We recommend the *benzodiazepines*—chlordiazepoxide (Librium, SK-Lygen), diazepam (Valium), oxazepam (Serax), clorazepate dipotassium (Tranxene), etc.—because they are:

a. specific in antianxiety action,
b. well tolerated,
c. generally safe both alone and with other medications (although CNS depression is a factor with some drugs, anesthetics, and alcohol; see Table 5),
d. essentially nonlethal in uncomplicated overdose,
e. rapid in onset of action,
f. not ordinarily strongly addicting (although they are abusable),
g. available for many routes of administration and
h. inexpensive.

In addition, their efficacy in control of certain acute seizures and in modulation of withdrawal symptoms makes them of considerable use to the physician.

Cautions:

a. Overuse of even a safe drug is usually a sign that the patient is in emotional difficulty and that there may be more useful ways for the physician to be of help.
b. IV dosage of diazepam should be undertaken carefully and slowly, since "push" administration can lead to respiratory arrest.

c. Oxazepam has the shortest half-life (six hours), is least hepatotoxic, and has not been reported to increase hostility via "paradoxical rage," as have some other benzodiazepines.

d. These anxiolytics may remove a veneer of anxiety to reveal an underlying depression; the physician should try to discern depression beforehand, lest the patient take several doses and encounter serious depressive symptoms or suicidal ideation.

e. Meprobamate (Miltown, Equanil, Sk-Bamate) is highly addicting. Withdrawal seizures have been reported in patients taking little more than routine doses.

III.D: OTHER COMMONLY USED DRUGS

1. Stimulants

a. are primarily amphetamines and methylphenidate;

b. have little use in adult psychiatry;

c. are short-term stimulants, not mood elevators;

d. should be used only in cases medically requiring alerting and in the occasional child who shows a true (neuropsychiatrically diagnosed) hyperactivity syndrome related to minimal brain dysfunction and responsive to the drug.

2. Sleeping Medications

a. One rarely needs anything stronger than flurazepam (Dalmane) 15–30 mg. H.S., or even the soporific side effect of psychotropic medications already prescribed.

b. Barbiturates and most other potent soporifics tend to suppress needed REM sleep (unlike the benzodiazepines) and may interfere with the activity of psychotropic medications.

3. Antiparkinsonian Preparations

a. Include benztropine mesylate (Cogentin) and other artificial antispasmotics such as trihexyphenidyl (Artane, Tremin); do not include L-DOPA;

b. Are of use to psychiatry in the control of extrapyramidal side effects of neuroleptic medication (see *Neuroleptics* above) such as:

    i. intention tremor,

    ii. body rigidity,

    iii. mask facies,

    iv. dysarthria and drooling,

    v. akathisia (uncontrollable restlessness or shuffling of feet: "Can't sit still"),

    vi. acute dystonia (see *Emergencies* section, page 15).

c. Are not useful for tardive dyskinesia.

d. Patients may complain when these drugs are discontinued even though the physician sees no need for them. Such a complaint may arise because

    i. the patient is telling the physician that he or she does not like the doctor's meddling with his medication, *or*

    ii. the medication is treating an akathisia or other subtle effect (perhaps primary parkinsonism) which is perceived by the patient but not noticeable to the physician.

e. Effective dose range is usually low; about 2–6 mg./day for benztropine, 4–12 mg./day for trihexyphenidyl.

f. Overdoses of these and other anticholinergic drugs may be treated with parenteral physostigmine, which effectively antagonizes the anticholinergic activity, in doses of 1 to 4 mg. IM or IV.

Amantadine (Symmetrel) is not anticholinergic, is not hepatically metabolized, and may be of use in refractory parkinsonian symptoms. Tolerance does develop and long-term use is not recommended.

A number of other drugs may be seen on specialized psychiatric units and in conjunction with other specialties, especially neurology, including phenytoin, other anticonvulsants, certain progesterone-like drugs and the like. These should by and large be reserved for use in such specialized areas as control of aggression, learning disabilities, cyclical or seizure-like syndromes, etc., and are of little everyday interest to the non-psychiatric physician.

III.E: INAPPROPRIATE PRESCRIPTION OF PSYCHOTROPIC MEDICATIONS

1. Neuroleptics

    a. are not anxiolytics and should not be substituted for the "minor tranquilizers";

    b. are not primarily sedatives and should not be used to quiet agitated patients unless the cause of the agitation is a neuroleptic-responsive psychosis;

    c. are CNS toxic and should therefore be cautiously used in the elderly, in seizure disorders, in withdrawal states, and in any organic CNS condition.

2. Lithium

    a. is not a panacea;

    b. should not be used as sole therapy for depression without careful psychiatric evaluation of the condition and evidence that the patient is a "lithium responder."

3. Antidepressants

    a. are often not what the name implies. They are useless and may be dangerous if given for just any depression, such as situational reactions, ordinary "blues," routine early-life depressions, etc.

    b. are not harmless. They can be lethal in overdose and toxic at routine doses. Physostigmine 1–4 mg. IM or IV reverses anticholinergic toxic effects. Repeat as needed.

    c. do not act quickly. You cannot give antidepressants for

depression in the same way that one gives anxiolytics for anxiety or antibiotics for infection.

4. Anxiolytics ("Minor Tranquilizers")

   a. are not panaceas. They should be used as temporary escape valves, not chronic coping mechanisms, if there are other ways to approach the symptoms.
   b. are not antipsychotic. They will not alleviate functional psychosis or be active against other psychoses, unless the psychosis is related to anxiety. These drugs do not affect thought disorder. They may, however, be useful in control of anxiety accompanying such syndromes.
   c. may rarely impair impulse control much as does ethanol.

5. Stimulants

   a. are not antidepressants;
   b. can produce paranoid psychosis at "therapeutic" levels, and especially with chronic use or abuse.

6. Sleeping Medications

don't give helpful sleep unless they promise REM sleep, or at least are short-enough-acting that they leave time for natural sleep before the patient awakens.

7. Antiparkinsonians

are not tranquilizers or otherwise significantly psychoactive, although they may become an emotionally important part of the patient's regimen or treat subtle, physician-unnoticed side effects.

8. Less is More

   a. There is little reason for mixing more than one medication from any of the mentioned major categories, and usually little reason for giving more than one or two meds in all.

TABLE 5: Common Drug Interactions (N.B.: * = Critical interaction)

Drug #1	Drug/Group #2	Potential Effect
Alcohol (see other drugs below)	*antipsychotics, tricyclic antidepressants, anxiolytics, CNS depressants, MAO inhibitors	*increased CNS depression; increased absorption of (at least) benzodiazepines
"	*Salicylates	*GI bleeding
Amphetamines	antipsychotics, benzodiazepines	possible decreased effect of #2
"	tricyclic antidepressants	possible increased effect of #2
"	*MAO inhibitors	*possible hypertensive crisis
Anesthetics	antipsychotics, tricyclics, CNS depressants, alcohol	increased CNS depression
Anticholinergics	antipsychotics, antiparkinsonians, tricyclics	increased anticholinergic activity (potential paralytic ileus, urinary retention)
Anticoagulants	tricyclics	increased anticoagulant effect with dicumerol
"	antipsychotics, tricyclic antidepressants	possible decreased anticoagulant effect, especially with heparin and antipsychotics
Antidiabetics	phenothiazines, tricyclic antidepressants	increased effect of antidiabetic except for chlorpromazine, which may antagonize it
Antiparkinsonians	phenothiazines	reduced blood levels of phenothiazine
"	antipsychotics, antidepressants	additive anticholinergic effects
Anxiolytics, benzodiazepines	*alcohol	*increased CNS depression
	CNS depressants, narcotic analgesics	increased CNS depression

Drug #1	Drug/Group #2	Potential Effect
Anxiolytics, meprobamate	*alcohol	*CNS depression
"	MAO inhibitors, CNS depressants, pheno-thiazines	increased CNS depression
Butyrophenones	Methyldopa	increased haloperidol toxicity
"	epinephrine	blocked hypertensive action of #2
"	lithium	increased lithium toxicity
Diuretics	lithium	lithium toxicity
"	phenothiazines	hypotension
"	tricyclics	Generally increased toxic effects of psychoactive drugs, depending on diuretic used.
Levodopa	antipsychotics, phenytoin, antiparkinsonians	? increased antidepressant effect, increased CNS depression
"	MAO inhibitors	decreased effect of Levodopa
Lithium carbonate	haloperidol	hypertensive crisis
"	tricyclic antidepressants	increased lithium toxicity
"	sodium depleting diuretics	possible increased antidepressant effect
		increased lithium toxicity
MAO inhibitors	*tricyclics, levodopa, narcotic analgesics, epinephrine, methylphenidate, tyramine (foods and beverages), amphetamines, other MAOI's, some alcohols	*hypertensive crisis, possible convulsions and coma
"	dextromethorphan	possible hyperthermia
"	antidiabetics	decreased effectiveness of antidiabetics

"	meperidine	*possible hypotensive or hypertensive crisis, severe CNS depression
"	CNS depressants, antiparkinsonians	increased depressant and anticholinergic effects
"	Anesthetics, general and spinal	increased CNS depression; possible hypotension
Narcotic analgesics	antipsychotics, anxiolytics, CNS depressants	further CNS depression, antipsychotics may seemingly augment analgesic action of narcotics
Oral contraceptives	tricyclic antidepressants	decreased antidepressant effect
Phenothiazines	clonidine, guanethidine	decreased antihypertensive effect
"	epinephrine	blocked hypertensive effect of epinephrine
"	antiparkinsonians, barbiturates, ? lithium	decreased antipsychotic effect of phenothiazines
Phenytoin	anticoagulants	increased DPH (phenytoin) toxicity
"	antipsychotics, tricyclics	decreased anticonvulsant activity
Tricyclic antidepressants	thyroid preparations, methylphenidate, some phenothiazines	increased antidepressant effect; possible thyrotoxicity with thyroid preparations
"	alcohol, barbiturates, oral contraceptives	decreased antidepressant effect
"	*MAO inhibitors	*hyperpyrexia, convulsion, hypertensive crisis
"	antiparkinsonians	increased anticholinergic effect
"	*epinephrine, other sympathomimetic (adrenergic) agents	*possible hypertensive crisis
"	guanethidine, clonidine, methyldopa	decreased antihypertensive effect; especially guanethidine

b. With the exception of lithium and some of the anxiolytics and antiparkinsonians, all of the commonly used medications cited can be given in once-daily doses. There are a few patients in whom brief periods of toxicity may occur if meds are given all at once, especially some elderly patients.

c. For long-term medication patients, especially those taking neuroleptics, try to achieve the lowest effective dose.

9. In the Beginning, Give Enough

Monitor for side effects and use good clinical judgment concerning possibilities of adverse reactions. However, don't make the dual error of exposing the patient to the drugs on the one hand but not giving sufficient medication to allow maximal chance of remission of symptoms.

10. Children

should not be given neuroleptic or antidepressant medication (or perhaps even methylphenidate) without consultation with someone expert in child psychiatry.

III.F: USE OF PSYCHOTROPIC DRUGS IN PREGNANT AND NURSING WOMEN

There is little firm evidence that therapeutic doses of psychotropic drugs result in significant damage to the embryo or fetus. There are, however, findings of teratology and spontaneous abortion in research involving very large doses of many psychotropics in some animal models (usually rodent), as well as rare anecdotal reports of complications in humans. These, and the fact that definitive human research is presently impossible to design, have lead to the vague general *caveats* found in the prescribing information for all psychotropic medications and in the *AMA Drug Evaluations*. See Table 6 for more information.

As for any treatment decision, potential benefits must be

weighed against possible detriments. Mitigating factors should be discussed with the patient and documented in the chart. In many cases, prescriptions can be postponed until pregnancy is ruled out or the first 60 days of gestation have passed. When clinically indicated, conservative drug therapy is virtually always without incident, except perhaps in the case of lithium (see Table 6).

TABLE 6: Drugs in Pregnancy and Nursing

Drug or Group	Teratology First Trimester	Cross Placenta	Late Fetal and Neonatal	Amount in Milk of Mother
Phenothiazines*	Small rodents with *large* doses; no good human evidence for teratology.	yes	Hepatotoxic and may cause jaundice or hyperbilirubinemia; possible respiratory depression or extra-pyramidal symptoms.	Trace.
Haloperidol, Thioxanthenes*	Same as Phenothiazines.	yes	Probably same as Phenothiazines.	Small amounts; unknown significance.
Tricyclic Antidepressants	Probably same as Phenothiazines, although slight implication for limb reduction.	yes	Possible respiratory or cardiac distress.	None known.
Benzodiazepines (diazepam chlordiazepoxide, oxazepam)	Laboratory animals with *large* doses; no good human evidence. Oral clefts in rare reports.	yes	Respiratory distress in large doses. Diazepam less so and is drug of choice in intrauterine asphyxiation.	Small amounts.

Meprobamate	Probably same as Benzodiazepines.	yes	Respiratory distress in large doses. Watch for abstinence syndrome in newborn.	Appreciable amounts.
Barbiturates	Probably same as Phenothiazines.	yes	Respiratory depression. Abstinence syndrome in addicts.	Small amounts.
Lithium	Laboratory animals with large doses. Possibly rarely in humans (especially cardiovascular).	yes	No known effects.	Appreciable. Mothers on Lithium should not nurse, though no toxicity case has been reported.

NOTE: Loxapine succinate (Loxitane) and molindone (Moban), both fairly new non-phenothiazine neuroleptics, have not had sufficient animal or human testing to establish presence or absence of human embryotoxicity or significant amounts in mothers' milk.

IV Other Organic Therapies

IV.A: ELECTROCONVULSIVE THERAPY (ECT)

1. ECT is primarily specific for severe depression of the types generally discussed as appropriate for antidepressant medication (see *Depression* and *Medication* sections). It is not usually indicated for other conditions, such as minor depressions, other affective disorders, and the functional psychoses (except for certain specifically refractory cases of schizophrenia).
2. Onset of action is rapid—days as opposed to the weeks of pharmacologic approaches. This can be life-saving in potentially suicidal situations.
3. The success rate is similar to that of the tricyclic medications, although
   a. ECT may address a slightly different group of patients, and
   b. may be used after failure of antidepressant drug therapy.
4. ECT itself is safe:
   a. Used appropriately, it has fewer serious side effects than the tricyclic antidepressants.
   b. Anesthesia and striatal muscle relaxants increase comfort and patient acceptance; however, they introduce additional dangers. The physician must be certain of his anesthesiological abilities or, better, have a specialized consultant in attendance.
   c. ECT may be given without anesthetic, thus eliminating

the inherent dangers of general anesthesia and succinylcholine-like relaxants, but adding the traumata of anticipation and generalized convulsion. Most centers use anesthetic.

d. There is a period of confusion following treatment, much like that following a grand mal seizure.

   i. This may be cumulative over the course of weeks of treatment.

   ii. Orientation and support by the unit staff help alleviate much of this confusion.

   iii. The patient's sensorium only very rarely suffers any lasting, measurable deficit.

e. The therapeutic effect is not directly related to the electricity used, hence the inaccuracy of the term "shock treatment." The skull and its attendant structures are insulators, so that most of the electrical current used passes through the subcutaneous fluid and out via the receiving electrode, with only a small amount reaching the surface of the brain and depolarizing it sufficiently to cause a convulsion.

5. Eight to 15 treatments, at two- or three-day intervals, are a complete course.

a. More treatments rarely increase chances of remission.

b. Fewer treatments, even though they may seem acutely effective, are associated with short-lived remission and later relapse.

6. ECT is often maligned because of

a. misunderstanding within the lay public,

b. probable overuse in the past, and

c. inappropriate use.

d. Stories of lasting intellectual deterioration, etc., if factual, are frequently attributable to

   i. inordinately large numbers of treatments over time,

   ii. accompanying pharmacologic or other treatment,

   iii. the natural course of a patient's disease, or

   iv. the sometimes striking effects of chronic institutionalization.

IV.B: MEGAVITAMIN TREATMENT

Although the use of large doses of vitamins and some other dietary supplements in the treatment of schizophrenia was publicized some years ago, there is no well-controlled study of such treatments which shows significant benefit to psychotic patients. In addition, studies of antipsychotic medication *versus* antipsychotic medication plus megavitamins have indicated no increase in treatment success.

IV.C: DIETARY TREATMENTS

Various kinds of diets have been proposed. Some (such as the gluten-free diet) have some basis in our current level of theoretical knowledge regarding the biochemical bases of schizophrenia and other severe mental illness. Other diets attempt to address the possibility of food allergens. Unfortunately, there is little or no good evidence for the efficacy of such diets, beyond the need for nutritionally balanced meals, as major components of treatment of the psychoses. Studies are continuing, however, and the existence of subtypes of the major psychiatric diagnoses which may be amenable to dietary treatment is a matter for future consideration.

IV.D: PSYCHOSURGICAL APPROACHES

These approaches, including leucotomy, have little or no place in the general treatment of the disorders discussed in this text. Precise stereotaxic procedures have occasionally been of use in severe and refractory neurological sequelae of medication reactions (e.g., tardive dyskinesia) and there is some evidence for their potential in some rare neuropsychiatric conditions.

v Psychotherapies

V.A: INDIVIDUAL THERAPY

There are a number of levels of individual psychotherapeutic treatment which may be useful within the medical setting. The first level is that of ordinary humane treatment, careful explanation of procedures, pleasant and understanding ward environment, and the like. These measures may go a long way toward alleviation of the fears and other discomforts felt by patients of any type, medical/surgical or psychiatric. More formal descriptions of individual therapies are listed below:

1. In *counseling,* the physician or other knowledgeable person talks with the patient in an *educational* way, sharing information and advice.
2. In *supportive therapy,* the physician or other therapist does more listening than talking, attempting to understand the patient's feelings and support him within the situation in which he finds himself. This may include a passive acceptance of the patient's feelings about his illness or other issues, or support for a decision which the patient has made regarding some aspect of his life (including his medical treatment). It implies empathy, concern, and "I'm on your side." Supportive therapy does not include challenges to decisions that the patient has already made, major confrontations, active attempts at educating the patient, or "orders." Supportive therapy may last for only a few minutes or be an ongoing process.
3. *Insight-oriented therapies* take a different approach. All such therapies have in common an attempt to make the patient more aware of emotional conditions within himself, usually by promoting self-discovery of these rather

than by direct statement or education. This emotional information may then be used by the patient to better understand himself and, if he chooses, to use that understanding within an organized program of personal change. Insight may be gained rapidly or very slowly, and may take months of searching and preparation. Once the insight is gained, the patient may use it or rebury it, depending upon the balance between his need for change (i.e., his discomfort), and his fears of change and the discomfort produced by the revealing of insight which had been previously unavailable to him. *Psychoanalytic therapy* is a refinement of insight-oriented therapy which shifts the focus from repressed events and feelings to the therapeutic relationship itself. Eventually, in psychoanalysis, the relationship between the therapist and the patient (transference and countertransference) becomes not only the matrix for treatment but an analyzable representation of the patient's psychodynamic core.

4. *Behavioral therapies* differ from most of the above in that they are particularly symptom-oriented and usually do not require an interpersonal relationship between therapist and patient, although this may develop and may be helpful. Utilizing the principle of reward for appropriate behavior and/or punishment (or withholding of reward) for inappropriate behavior, this approach has been used in a wide variety of situations with varying results. Highly structured programs with well-controlled "conditioning paradigms" are very successful in changing *behavior*. The probability of changes in underlying signs and symptoms varies considerably among diagnoses and treatment settings.

5. The *existential* approaches have to do with philosophy of life and with discovery or acceptance of one's place within one's universe. Such activities as the various Yogas and Transcendental Meditation, although commonly denying that they represent psychotherapies, may be of benefit. It should be noted that although patient reports of subjective improvement are common, controlled

studies are few and the use of these approaches for certain specific symptoms (e.g., phobias, hypertension) has yielded conflicting data.

6. *Biofeedback* is primarily a behavioral therapy, although it necessarily involves a relaxation not unlike some of the existential approaches. In this form of treatment, the patient is made aware of the presence of, and changes in, certain of his physical characteristics, sometimes characteristics which are not ordinarily accessible to consciousness (e.g., hand temperature, *frontalis* tension). By postulating a relationship between the characteristic which is "fed back" and the symptom or illness to be treated, control over the characteristic may lead to alleviation of the symptom. Studies of degree and duration of relief, as well as of the appropriateness of associating a given target characteristic with a given symptom or illness, are inconclusive and sometimes conflicting.

V.B: COUPLE AND FAMILY THERAPY

Therapy with couples and families, like most other forms of therapy described herein, requires a strong working alliance and a willingness on the part of the participants to communicate clearly, so that the therapist is better able to achieve an understanding of the structure and function of the participants' lives together. Unlike individual therapy, in the case of couple and family therapy the "patient" is more the marital dyad or the entire family than any individual within the pair or group. This means that the techniques of counseling, support or insight seen in individual therapy are now applied to the couple's *relationship* or the family's *system* rather than to individuals, as the therapist becomes a catalyst for communication and exploration of problems which are brought to the office.

Temptations to "take sides," to "referee" or to identify a particular member of the couple or family as "sick" or "the real patient" should be avoided in most kinds of couple and family treatment. Symptoms, responsibility, power in the relationship, and the like are usually carefully balanced among the members. Well-meaning but premature attempts at what may on the surface appear to be logical intervention often lead to little assistance with the real problems or, worse, to a destructive influence on an already precariously balanced, highly complex set of relationships.

V.C: GROUP THERAPY

As in the case of individual therapy, a number of approaches may be useful. Primarily, the use of group treatment allows for a diffusing of emotions and therefore a "defusing" of their impact on the patient. Learning that others have problems similar to one's own, learning to trust others and share oneself with them, and learning that others may be a source of help and support are all important characteristics of group therapy. In addition, observations or insights which come from more than one person—especially from one's peers—may be at once more difficult for the patient to avoid and easier for him to accept. Finally, the experience of interacting in the group setting on a regular basis serves as a model for other social interactions and can be a useful vehicle for testing and patterning, in a safe setting, some new behaviors and coping mechanisms which the patient may later wish to incorporate into his daily life.

Groups may be quite specific and goal-oriented, as with those designed for "anorgasmic" women or phobic air travelers. Other groups may be more general and supportive in nature, such as regular social get-togethers for chronic psychiatric outpatients, who may benefit from the social interaction of being with others while at the same time enjoying attention and relief from boarding home routine. Still other groups may be quite insight-oriented, using the group setting over a long period of time to promote more generalized personal growth through a series of insights not unlike intensive individual therapy.

The therapist in a group situation faces a number of tasks which are different from those of individual treatment. On the one hand, he has the assistance of the group members, and often of a co-therapist, in observing characteristics of the members, supporting them, and communicating information or interpretations, as appropriate. On the other hand, the amount of information and number of things which need to be observed and understood increase dramatically in the group setting when compared to individual therapy.

V.D: CRISIS THERAPY

Treatment of the patient in acute emotional crisis, perhaps crisis precipitated by acute physical trauma or loss, is an especially important area. This is a situation which is likely to present to the treating physician and which cannot (or should not) often be referred to one's psychiatric colleagues for more definitive handling the next day or the next week. One may be faced with the family of an accident victim, a couple who have just had a violent argument, a patient who is terrified of a surgical procedure which is scheduled for the next day, or a patient with whom one must discuss the prospect of terminal illness. Some of these are situations in which the physician becomes involved because he is the emergency contact. Others are situations in which the physician is sought out because he is the patient's "doctor," someone known to the patient (as opposed to an unknown psychiatrist or social worker), and/or because he is the person who has done the "laying on of hands."

First, *listen*. Although you may have feelings of your own that you want to express, you may wish to avoid the situation, or you may feel that your talking will help things considerably, remember that it is *the patient's* crisis. If no words or feelings are forthcoming from the patient, let him or her know that you want to understand and that you hope the patient will share his feelings with you when he is ready. Of course, in many situations words and feelings will pour out of everyone at once. Still, listen, at least for a few moments. If the situation is one which requires a particular action, such as consent for surgery, understanding of medical instructions, or psychiatric evaluation, let your quiet control of yourself begin to influence the setting in such a way as to promote de-escalation of the clamor, confusion, and apprehension. This firm but kind control, coupled with the need to complete a specific task at hand, may be very helpful.

Crises are by definition temporary. A person cannot remain in a crisis for very long; however, the way in which he or she handles the situation, perhaps with your guidance, will determine which of three possible outcomes is finally attained:

a. chronic regression to a less mature, less adaptive lifestyle;

b. restabilization at about the same level of adaptation and coping; or

c. emergence of a more mature, more adaptive, and generally more comfortable way of dealing with life, perhaps as a result of confidence gained by successfully coping with the just-passed crisis.

V.E: INPATIENT MILIEU AND PARTIAL HOSPITALIZATION

The setting in which the psychiatric patient who requires hospitalization is treated is an important part of his treatment and can be considered a form of therapy. Such a ward may be very close to other hospital units, denoting acceptance of psychiatric treatment as a part of overall care, or it may be separate from them because of special facility requirements or old stereotypes. In any event, the psychiatric ward

a. should be geared for the professional treatment of patients by specially-trained staff;

b. should be unlocked;

c. should offer a pleasant, open, community atmosphere commensurate with the personal rights and ambulatory nature of the patients;

d. must have facilities and staff available for milieu, group, occupational, and recreational therapies.

Individualized programs for each patient should be formulated, going beyond routine organic therapies and aiming toward successful re-entry into the family and community.

Certain patients may benefit from therapy programs which are neither as restrictive (and expensive) as inpatient care nor as unstructured as outpatient status. Such patients may require *partial hospitalization,* perhaps for several hours per day. In these programs, the emphasis should be on an active course of treatment leading to resocialization and confidence in one's ability to live away from the institution. This may take several weeks or months but should always be seen as the goal of a dynamic process. Partial hospitalization facilities should not be confused with some other programs in which custodial care, rather than progress, may be the primary orientation.

VI Psychological Testing

The various forms of psychological testing should not be used as substitutes for personal contact with the patient. However, they can be of considerable use in a number of psychiatric and medical situations. We recommend that the physician become familiar with the people in his institution or community who do psychological testing. He should also know what kinds of tests are available and how one actually orders them. We further recommend that the physician pay attention to test results and to the comments of the psychologist.

VI.A: TESTS OF ORGANIC FUNCTIONING, INCLUDING INTELLIGENCE

Whether and how well the cerebrum and its attendant structures are functioning are important in a variety of situations (the subject of the testing of other parts of the CNS and of the peripheral nervous system shall be left to neurological texts). Determination of baseline values of organic damage or intellectual functioning should especially be done when one is contemplating treatment designed to alleviate deficits in these areas, or procedures which may alter such functions. The new stroke patient; patients being considered for neurosurgery; patients being considered for long-duration surgery (especially cardiovascular procedures and those involving CNS hemodynamics); patients suffering severe intoxications, overdoses, or other sources of anoxia; psychiatric patients (especially those with undetermined diagnoses and "new" symptoms), and the like are all candidates for baseline organic testing. In appropriate hands, such tests may also be used in diagnosis and in treatment planning.

Common tests which are administered to test organic function include

a. The Bender-Gestalt (in which the patient reproduces drawings of simple two-dimensional patterns),
b. The Halstead-Reitan Battery and the Luria-Nebraska Neuropsychological Battery (which comprehensively address motor, sensory, intellectual, and language abilities), and
c. The Eisenson Test of Aphasia (an orally administered test of language function).
d. In addition, certain portions of the Wechsler Adult Intelligence Scale (WAIS) and similar tests may give information regarding organic CNS function.

"Intelligence tests," such as the WAIS, involve a series of parts which are statistically associated with characteristics of that which the test calls "intelligence" (ability to assimilate, recall, and manipulate information, in most instances). The tests are generally divided into *verbal* (written and spoken words and numbers) and *performance* (spatial manipulation and other nonverbal skills) portions, with the total score sometimes expressed as an "intelligence quotient" ("IQ").

The psychologist will, in his discussion of the results, compare various portions of the tests in order to estimate such things as the presence of higher intelligence than verbal skills might indicate, or the presence of considerable verbal skills with an impaired ability to translate them into usable activity. Of course, considerations such as social and educational background, cultural differences, and language difficulties must be considered. Results of these and other psychological tests should never be considered in the absence of other information, preferably personally obtained, about the patient.

VI.B: EMOTIONAL TESTS, OBJECTIVE AND PROJECTIVE

Although not entirely separate from the above, there are a wide variety of tests available which purport to give the examiner a great deal of information about a patient's psychological makeup with a minimum of time and invasiveness. *Objective* tests

a. are well standardized,
b. are usually written,
c. require specific yes-no or multiple-choice answers,
d. yield quantifiable information,
e. are often more replicable than the alternatives below, and
f. can often be interpreted, at least in a cursory fashion, by trained technicians or computers.

Examples of such tests include the Minnesota Multiphasic Personality Inventory (MMPI) and the "16 PF."
Projective tests

a. allow greater choice of response from the subject,
b. require that clinical inference be made by the person evaluating the results, and
c. purport to extrapolate nuances of the subject's responses to ambivalent situations into important psychological information about him or her.

For example, the subject's responses to the various "inkblots" of the Rorschach test may, in appropriate professional hands, give information about his personality. The Thematic Apperception Test (TAT) is similar in that it requires the subject to interpret and comment upon pictures purposely designed to be ambiguous. Sentence completion tests and similar instruments take advantage of immediate responses to brief vignettes (e.g., *"If I saw my best friend drowning, I would _____."*).

Tests which require performance by the subject, such as the Draw-a-Person, House-Tree-Person (H-T-P), and Draw-a-Family tests, may give information about the subject's image of himself and his perception of his place in his family or universe. Such drawing tests are most often used with children, sometimes as part of testing for levels of intellectual functioning. Evaluation of a patient's unrequested art work, letters, compositions, poems, etc., may also be considered projective testing since projective testing takes advantage of the idea that *the patient will endow persons or things outside himself with characteristics which are related to his own psychological makeup.*

VII Psychosomatic Medicine

> "It is more important to know what sort of person has a disease than to know what sort of disease a person has."
>
> —Hippocrates

Psychosomatic disease is *common*. Some 20 percent of all patients seen by family doctors and 70 percent of patients with chronic disease have psychosomatic symptoms as major components of their illness.

It should be remembered that

1. Chronic emotional or psychosomatic symptomatology may lead to organic pathology and concomitant disability.
2. Psychosomatic diagnoses are unpopular with patients and physicians. The patient may be left with a loss of self-image if no "organic disease" is present. Office visits tend to take more of the physician's time and patience, sometimes with less professional reward.

VII.A: ETIOLOGIC SCHEMATA

There are four basic processes through which emotions may effect physical symptoms and/or organic pathology.

1. Emotions → Symptoms (Direct effect).
   Examples: Tears accompanying grief, fainting at the sight of blood.
2. Emotions → Mediating Behaviors → Symptoms.
   Examples: Anorexia nervosa, aerophagia (air swallowing).
3. Physical or emotional symptoms → Psychological reactions → More Symptoms.

Examples: Exertional angina produces anxiety which may perpetuate pain, elevate blood pressure, and increase risk of arrhythmias in a patient with severe coronary artery disease; *or* an anxious patient fears "going crazy" or being "out of control," leading to escalated anxiety ("anxiety reaction").

4. Emotional Symptoms → Nonpsychological mediators → Other Symptoms.

   Example: Depressed patient taking tricyclic medication complains of blurry vision.

VII.B: EVALUATION OF PATIENTS WITH PSYCHOSOMATIC SYMPTOMS

1. Initial approach to the patient may be of therapeutic value if the physician is perceived as warm, honest, and reassuring.
2. Taking a good history and completing a mental status exam will save time in the long run.
3. Particularly appropriate to the clarification of psychosomatic components of symptoms are:

   a. The patient's *affect* as he relates the history.

      Example: The *"belle indifférence"* of hysterical symptoms.

   b. Recently diagnosed asymptomatic disease.

      Example: A newly diagnosed hypertensive patient who experiences esophageal reflux, then hyperventilates and experiences palpitations.

   c. Life changes and social history. Patients with a recent history of social or family stress will very often experience a change of health status (see Table 7).

Changes in health status tend to cluster about significant life changes.

   d. Family history
      i. "Medical portion": family members with disease.

TABLE 7: Life Changes Related to Emotional and/or Psychophysiological Symptoms*

Event	Scale of Impact†
Death of spouse	100
Divorce	73
Jail term	63
Death of close family member	63
Personal injury, illness	53
Marriage	50
Fired from work	47
Retirement	45
Pregnancy	40
New family member (child, sibling)	39
Death of close friend	37
Child leaving home to begin adult life	29
Beginning or ending schooling	26
Wife starts or stops working	26
Change in work conditions, residence, school	20
Holidays, vacations	12–13

* Abbreviated from Holmes, T. H. and Rahe, R. H. "The social adjustment rating scale." *J. Psychosom. Res.* 11:213, 1967.

† Events experienced over one year which total 200 or more (including stresses listed in the more complete list) are associated with significant physical and/or emotional disease in a large majority of individuals.

> *Example:* "Cancer scare" in patients with a strong family history of cancer.

  ii. "Social portion": patient's perception of an interaction between other family members.

> *Example:* A child's asthmatic symptoms which are correlated with the parents' marital difficulties.

  iii. "Anniversary phenomena."

> *Example:* An entertainer who "coincidentally" becomes severely ill almost exactly one year after the death of his mother.

4. Physical examination.

  a. Physical examination may be of *therapeutic value* as reassurance to the patient.

    b. Confer with the patient after the examination. Be honest with yourself and the patient. If you have not made a diagnosis, do not offer one.

    c. Explain in understandable terms the diagnostic rationale for tests that you have planned for the patient. Offer reassurance if a diagnostic procedure will be unfamiliar or uncomfortable.

    d. If no gross physical abnormalities related to symptoms can be found, present this to the patient in a reassuring fashion. Be careful not to phrase your words to imply that the patient "is a crock" or that the symptoms are "all in his head."

Psychosomatic symptoms are real. They are not imagined nor are they under voluntary control of the patient.

VII.C: TREATMENT

Among the elements of treatment are:

1. Rapport—supportive, concerned, and professional—and reassurance.
2. Patient education that the psyche can produce symptoms or even organic disease through physiological mediators.
   Example: Vagal stimulation of gastric acid secretion in patients with duodenal ulcer disease.
3. Brief explanation of diagnostic rationale, therapeutic modalities and therapeutic goals.
4. Definitive treatment should be aimed at the emotional source of the symptoms (e.g., depression) whenever possible.
5. Symptomatic medical treatment may be useful or palliative, but in most patients should not be a substitute for definitive, psychiatrically-oriented intervention (see *Psychotherapies*).
6. Often the patient may be asked to "Carry on in spite of the symptoms."
   Example: "I understand that your work makes you feel

nauseous; but while we're working to find the cause, you still need to earn a living."

Referral to a Psychiatrist

The physician should become familiar with sources of psychiatric consultation and treatment within the medical center or community. Medical schools, community mental health centers, and county medical associations may be of help.

Physicians as well as patients may harbor unrecognized feelings of suspiciousness toward psychiatry. Attitudes such as these, and feelings that a patient is being "dumped" onto the psychiatrist or other mental health professional, are easily communicated to the patient and can seriously undermine the potential usefulness of the referral. The psychiatrist should be considered a medical specialist whom you are asking for expert assistance, just as you would any other specialist.

When discussing the referral with the patient, be honest and frank, but supportive. Do not "threaten" the patient with psychiatric referral or try to "trick him into it." Simply tell the patient that his or her symptoms may have emotional concomitants and that the psychiatrist's knowledge and experience may be of help in understanding these components and alleviating their effects.

Both physician and patient should consider psychiatric referral much as any other referral; that is, as the use of a specialist whose additional knowledge of his field may be helpful to the patient.

(NOTE: For specific reference to medical conditions with important psychophysiologic concomitants, the reader is referred to Wittkower, E. D. and Warnes, H. (eds.): *Psychosomatic Medicine: Its Clinical Implications*. Hagerstown, MD: Medical Department, Harper & Row, 1977.)

VIII Special Patient Populations

VIII.A: INFANTS

Birth is not too early a time for the physician to begin his concern for the psychological health of his or her patient. Situations which put the infant at risk for emotional or developmental problems start even earlier, in the genetic makeup and prenatal environment, and continue with opportunities for obstetrical complications, perinatal distress and congenital defects. Even the small infant seems to have an innate "temperament" which influences his reactions and adaptations to his environment. Early recognition of such risk factors and temperaments, as well as recognition of the condition of the family in which he will be raised, is important in the prediction and prevention of such problems as maternal rejection or depression, failure to thrive, and developmental lags which, in turn, place the infant at risk for even more problems later in childhood.

When an infant behaves outside that which the physician or experienced parent believes is normal, specialized consultation should be sought promptly in the form of a child psychiatrist or pediatric neurologist, or both. Developmental milestones give some information about the neurological and psychological maturation of the infant, within a fairly narrow range of "normality":

AGE	NORMAL ACCOMPLISHMENTS
Birth	APGAR rating; flexion of limbs; reaction to stimuli.
4–6 weeks	Smiles at mother.
6–8 weeks	Vocalizes when smiling.

12–16 weeks	Turns head to sound; holds objects (not just instinctive grasp).
20 weeks	Reaches for objects near self.
26 weeks	Transfers objects from hand to hand; sits; feeds self biscuit.
9–10 months	Creeps; helps dress by extending hand or foot; "pat-a-cake," "bye-bye" motions.
13 months	Walks without help; knows 2–3 words.
15 months	Feeds self and drinks holding own cup if given the opportunity; mouthing of objects decreases considerably.
21–24 months	Joins 2–3 words in phrases; usually dry during day.
36 months	Dresses self except for difficult parts; stands on one foot; usually dry all night.

VIII.B: CHILDREN

The child with emotional problems—or whose parents describe such problems—deserves special consideration. Our concern in earlier pages has been with adults, often in situations in which intervention by the family physician is appropriate and useful. At this time, then, let us extend the *caveat* begun in the *Infants* section above: When there is a problem which you recognize as serious, which does not promptly respond to treatment, or which continues to be uncomfortable for the child or the family after you feel it has been treated appropriately, seek specialized consultation. The concepts of careful assessment and early definitive treatment are as important in child psychiatry as in any other branch of medicine.

The child must be evaluated in the context of the system in which he lives. This includes the important concept that he or she is actively developing, growing physically and emotionally throughout whatever psychological disease process (or treatment) may be superimposed upon that development. Assessment of the family and other parts of that dynamic environment must be carried out; the child is never an isolated bundle of symptoms. The following are some syndromes that are likely to present in any hospital or office practice.

1. *Depression.* Depression can occur at any age in children, even in infancy. It may be characterized by hopelessness, helpless feelings, apathy, sadness, crying or suicidal thoughts. "Depressive equivalents," symptoms that mask underlying depression, may include running away, stealing, or a number of other behaviors. Depression may be quite serious, even life-threatening, as in the case of "anaclitic depression" related to profound loss. *Treatment* is best referred to a child psychiatrist. Management of the parent-child relationship may be helpful. Later, play therapy or other interventions can be used.

2. *"Hyperactivity."* Hyperactivity often means that someone—at home or at school—doesn't like what the child is doing. Complaints of this symptom should be carefully evaluated before the child is seen as a "patient" and especially before medication is prescribed. In neuropsychologically documented instances of organic CNS dysfunction, stimulants such as methylphenidate or dextroamphetamine have an "organizing" effect in many preadolescent patients; however, other diagnoses must be ruled out and other treatments considered in each case.

3. *Hospitalization.* The child with serious medical illness and/or need for hospitalization should be treated with gentle honesty and respect. Attention to fears of the hospital, of procedures, of what might happen to him, and of separation from home and parents should include discussions (with, not about, the child), anticipatory play and rehearsals, allowing special toys or objects brought from home, liberal visitation arrangements and the like. In some cases, the parents may avoid or deny the seriousness of the child's illness more than the child himself. Try not to add to the unknown, the ambiguous, or even to deceit by withholding valuable information and support.

4. *School phobia.* School phobia is often part of a system

in which the child is playing a part and must maintain a particular image (e.g., that of a fearful child). Treatment is usually successful, provided appropriate child/family counseling is available. The child should not be allowed to avoid school totally during treatment, even if this only means going to school and sitting outside the classroom for a brief period.

5. *Running away.* Running away may reflect a wide variety of difficulties, most often family related. Age, duration and distance of the first episode may predict future problems.

6. *Enuresis.* Enuresis may be treated as an individual, family, or even neurological problem, depending upon onset and symptoms. No matter what the cause, remember that the child is usually embarrassed and uncomfortable, especially if he or she is of school age. Methods which reduce symptoms in a non-punitive way (moisture alarms, low doses of imipramine) may be useful while exploring family or psychodynamic factors involved.

7. *Emergencies.* For the child, a point of emotional emergency is reached when parenting figures can no longer provide appropriate controls or when his anxiety can no longer be mastered without external control. The child's or the family's cry for help is usually loud, such as a suicide attempt or painful physical symptoms; however, the cry does not always point toward the psychological cause, as when somatic illness arises or when one member of the family develops symptoms in response to another's disturbance. Do your best to get him or her (and the family) some *help.*

Finally, to repeat a point made in the section on adult psychotropic medications: Psychiatric medications should be used in children only with great caution, and then usually by specialists in child psychiatry or neurology. This recommendation is not meant to demean the abilities of nonpsychiatric practitioners; rather, it reflects the many complexities of the field, as well as its unknowns.

VIII.C: ADOLESCENTS

The adolescent patient shows significant medical and psychiatric differences from the adult. He often has an adult physical body, and it is often quite healthy; however, his emotions are in a state of constant flux and maturation and are often under considerable stress. In general, the adolescent is faced with the task of dealing with the reawakening of early childhood conflicts which have lain dormant for many years. His physical and social changes bring these issues to the fore and make it imperative that they be handled in some fairly permanent manner in order to eventually establish a stable adulthood.

The adolescent is often struggling with two basic conflicts:

a. that of the wish to retain the advantages of childhood *vs.* his dislike for the feeling of immaturity, *and*
b. the wish for the stability of maturity *vs.* his fear of the responsibilities that adulthood entails.

The adolescent is often frightened that his or her developing adult controls will fail and that his baser parts will come out to overwhelm him or to harm others. He is in need of education about life, self, and the world around him. He seeks stimulation in order both to further his store of experiences and to alleviate the many discomforts which may be related to the issues noted above.

Although we do not advocate using the adolescent's special status to exempt him from responsibility for his actions (e.g., for antisocial behavior), or to explain away clearly deviant or psychopathologic behavior as "just a stage," psychiatric diagnosis during these years should be approached with some caution. Since both the psyche and the CNS are in the process of maturing, the entry of serious diagnoses in a permanent record such as the hospital or office chart should be done with some care.

The adolescent is particularly sensitive to physical and emotional loss. Loss of face (e.g., having to admit that he is wrong, or being even mildly shamed in front of his peer group), loss of body image (whether from acne or amputation), or loss of his picture of himself as a healthy, normal person can be devastating. The adolescent who must face a diagnosis of diabetes, for example, or one who is referred to a psychiatrist with symptoms of severe emotional discomfort, should receive special support aimed at feelings of failure and unworthiness. These feelings may be covered by a veneer of bravado or by physical, sometimes socially deviant, activity.

Of course, when treating adolescents or children, an effort should be made to continue schooling and social activity with as little interruption as possible. This may include the use of a special adolescent unit within the hospital, a situation which is highly recommended since it avoids the dual problems of

a. placing a person who is not yet ready for adulthood on an adult-oriented unit, *or*
b. placing on a children's unit a person who is struggling with issues related to becoming an adult.

VIII.D: THE ELDERLY

We have already touched upon issues regarding organic differences between the elderly and the young adult patient, such as the need for differing medication regimens, special physical environments, and the like. In this brief section we should like to make a plea for the treatment of the elderly as persons, rather than as "non-persons" or as "temporary persons" who are about to die. Within the limitations of physical ability— limitations which may be overestimated—the older person should be treated as just that, an older *person*. He or she will likely be happier with this arrangement and will almost certainly respond better to your medical or psychiatric interventions.

This attitude may include trying not to "infantilize" or "talk down to" the elderly. While many people readily accept the medical notion of "You're the doctor," older people may be acutely aware that you are their chronological and experiential junior. Unless this issue is appropriately handled, it can result in difficulties with communication and in the patient's not accepting your ideas or recommendations.

The subject of living conditions is another with which the younger and older sets occasionally have difficulty. Although it is sometimes unavoidable, most people who have been self-sufficient for years do not wish to feel useless and dependent. We encourage compromise between the reality of physical frailty and the patient's needs for autonomy and privacy. Examples of such sensitive areas include

    a. institutionalization,
    b. mandatory retirement policies, and
    c. denial of the senior citizen's sexuality.

As stressed in the previous pages, it is the physician's responsibility to find out about available resources which can assist with these concepts. You need not have the entire social service network of your community at your fingertips; however, know some good information numbers to call and do your best to personally help the patient make contact with the next person in the social assistance chain.

VIII.E: THE DYING PATIENT, HIS FAMILY, AND THE PATIENT FACING OTHER SEVERE LOSS

    a. The dying patient is not always an elderly patient.
    b. The dying patient is not always in crisis (although crises may often arise).
    c. The dying patient, like the elderly patient, is a <u>person</u> and will benefit considerably if treated accordingly.

1. The Patient

The well known "stages" of dying (which may not be so stereotyped as earlier thought) include denial, anger, bargaining, depression, and acceptance. These should be watched for in the terminally ill person, and the physician should supportively assist both patient and family in dealing with them.

Although in some instances the patient will request privacy for his emotional work, the doctor should from the outset take some initiative in discussing the patient's condition, listening to the patient's comments and feelings and conveying an honest attitude of availability and willingness to help. Although it is often said that some patients "don't want to know" or "can sense that they are going to die; the doctor doesn't have to tell them," these seem to us to be cruel and unnecessary positions for the physician to take. If the patient doesn't want you around or doesn't want to talk that day, let him tell you so himself after you have offered some of your time. And offer your time again soon.

The dying patient rarely wishes to be left completely alone for any significant length of time. The physician should guard against such things as subtle avoidance of the patient on rounds or forgetting to drop by the hospital just before the weekend starts, and should act against the ward staff's tendency to similarly shut off the patient. The physician should strive to answer questions which the patient may have and should try to anticipate those questions which have gone unasked.

Reasonable requests for considerations, such as discharge from the hospital in order to die at home or the putting of control of pain medication into the patient's own hands, should be carefully weighed and granted whenever possible. Strict adherence to hospital regulations, attempts by the physician and other staff to control the patient's treatment and environment, and instigation of "heroic measures" are often, like the forgetting of the patient on rounds, indicative of the physician's own concerns about death and about the patient's terminal condition. In this context, although your feelings may be natural ones, try not to allow them to interfere with good overall patient care.

It has been said that the patient who is aware that he is going to die and can experience the end of life in a conscious and useful way is more fortunate than the patient who dies suddenly and unexpectedly. We shall all experience death and shall hopefully have around us people who will help to make this a true statement.

2. The Family

The family of the dying patient deserve much the same attention and consideration as the patient himself. They are, at least initially, in crisis and the principles of crisis intervention apply. Further, they may benefit, and so indirectly may the patient, from your assistance in educating them about treatment of the dying person and from your being a model of a person for whom death does not hold quite so much threat or mystery.

The single most important thing to communicate to the family members is that they must themselves communicate. They must communicate with the patient, not isolate him or think that they are "protecting" him with what is more accurately a "conspiracy of silence." This time needs to be used by both the family and the patient for important activities of grief, as well as for the realistic arrangements that must be made. To waste the time on silence and avoidance can be tragic.

Communication must also be open within the family. All family members, including children, should be apprised of the situation as soon as possible. Discussions should be open and the atmosphere one that allows for expression of all feelings— sadness, despair, anger, frustration, relief—from all members of the family. Certain family members, especially children, will benefit tremendously from observation and participation in the feelings of others. An adult's outward show of "stiff upper lip" or "big boys don't cry" serves as a poor model for the child, who needs to learn appropriate ways of handling and releasing his emotions both now and throughout later life.

3. Other Loss Experiences

Just as dying is primarily a *loss,* so do other losses bring with them some characteristics of the dying or grieving person. The reader may have noted throughout this book the continuing thread that *awareness of physical or emotional infirmity is, without exception, looked upon by the patient as a personal loss and a statement of decreased self worth.* Many of the principles enumerated in the previous paragraphs on the dying patient and his family should be kept in mind when you are dealing with a patient who has lost a limb, his health, his personal appearance or perceived attractiveness, his feelings of stability or sanity, his sense of immortality (e.g., as commonly happens with one's first encounter with serious illness), his physical mobility, his vocational ability or ability to be autonomous and useful, or a sensory modality (sight, hearing, etc.). All of these must be considered for the complete medical and psychosocial treatment of the patient.

ix Glossary of Psychiatric Terms

NOTE: For definitions and descriptions of specific psychiatric illnesses and symptoms, the reader is referred to the current edition of the American Psychiatric Association's *Diagnostic and Statistical Manual.*

Abreaction. Discharge of painful emotions which were previously unconscious. Sometimes therapeutic (e.g., in resolution of grief).

Acting Out. Unconsciously expressing feelings, memories, or conflicts by means of one's physical behavior. Patients in psychotherapy may "act out" outside the therapist's office issues that are difficult to verbally express in treatment (e.g., an alcoholic patient who, because of anger and anxiety related to treatment, becomes intoxicated).

Addiction. Physical dependence, usually to a chemical substance, manifested by a potential for physiologic withdrawal symptoms.

Affect. Subjective feelings, usually pleasant or unpleasant, often with physiologic components such as blushing, perspiration, posture, or facial expression.

Affective Disorder. A broad concept which refers to disorders of affect or mood, including depression and manic states.

Akathisia. An extrapyramidal condition often related to neuroleptic medication, manifested by restlessness and a difficulty sitting or standing in one place ("can't sit still").

Ambivalence. Simultaneous existence of opposing feelings or impulses. Ubiquitous and normal unless it exists to such an extent that the individual becomes limited in his ability to, for example, make decisions or carry out reasonable daily activities.

Anaclitic. In psychiatry, describes dependence of an infant on its caregiver(s). "Anaclitic depression" is a severe deprivation syndrome which may occur in infants who are separated, physically or emotionally, from the mother.

Anhedonia. Inability or severe difficulty in experiencing pleasure.

Anorexia Nervosa. A severe and often life-threatening syndrome, most frequently seen in adolescent girls, in which marked emotional conflict results in morbid avoidance of food, marked weight loss, and often genital dysfunction (e.g., amenorrhea).

Anxiety. An affect experienced subjectively and physiologically as fear. It may result from an anticipation of real (emotional or physical) danger or may be "free floating," that is, apparently unconnected to conscious feelings of external threat.

Autism. Severely egocentric thinking, often to a psychotic extent. In child psychiatry, a symptom which describes marked withdrawal and closing off from the external world in favor of inner thoughts and self-stimulation. May be confused with retardation.

Autoerotic. Refers to self-gratification including, but not limited to, masturbation. Characteristic of infancy, but related behaviors and feelings continue throughout life.

Automatism/Automatic Behavior. Behavior which is apparently not controlled or influenced by conscious thought. May be purposeful or undirected.

Belle Indifférence. Apparent inappropriate lack of concern or anxiety seen in some patients with hysterical conversion symptoms.

Blocking. An interruption of thought or speech which prevents unconsciously conflictual material from being expressed.

Body Image. The sum of conscious and unconscious impressions which a person has of his own body. Includes attractiveness, health, etc.

Borderline State. A descriptive (not diagnostic) reference to symptoms which appear to be neither psychotic nor nonpsychotic. The condition is sometimes unstable and the patient may sometimes appear to be psychotic.

Bulimia/Polyphagia. Morbidly increased hunger or eating behavior.

Castration Anxiety. A major source of conflict during early development. Usually expressed in symbolic events related to losses (e.g., threats to bodily integrity, humiliation, loss of job).

Catalepsy. A trance-like state of diminished responsiveness.

Cataplexy. Loss of voluntary muscle tone.

Catatonia. Usually a state of postural rigidity, often involving "waxy flexibility." May also refer to some agitated, excited states.

Catharsis. The process of releasing repressed or suppressed material into consciousness, generally in a therapeutic context and usually accompanied by appropriate affect.

Cathexis. The investment of emotional energy in a mental representation of an idea, symbol, or object. Most commonly, emotional attachment to another person.

Character Disorder. Chronic, habitual, relatively inflexible behavior traits which are deeply rooted in early development and which limit optimal use of emotional energy. These disorders are frequently experienced by the individual without pain or discomfort ("ego-syntonic"). When socially acceptable and/or subclinical, such disorders may be described as "character neurosis."

Collective Unconscious. A basic term of Jungian theory referring to that part of the unconscious which is found in all people.

Compensation Neurosis. A descriptive (not diagnostic) term for some psychiatric disabilities which feature secondary gain. Not "malingering," in that compensation neurosis has a predominantly unconscious basis.

Complex. Related emotional characteristics which, although generally unconscious, interact to influence attitudes and behavior (e.g., inferiority complex).

Compulsion. The recurring, unwanted, intrusive urge to engage in some behavior. The behavior is symbolically related to unconscious conflict, although the relationship may not be overtly visible. Resisting compulsions leads to anxiety.

Confabulation. An unconscious filling in of gaps in memory or social conversation by imaginary but superficially related information. Most commonly seen in organic CNS deficit.

Conflict. Intrapsychic conflict is the result of conflict between opposing impulses and demands within the self (e.g., the attraction a child has for his opposite-sexed parent versus his fear of retaliation or loss of love from the same-sexed parent). Conflict can also occur between the wishes and needs of the self and the realities of the external world.

Conversion/Hysterical Conversion. Closely related terms which refer to the defusing of anxiety-provoking conflictual material by means of external expression which is unconsciously symbolic of the conflict.

Counterphobic. Refers to the seeking out and engaging in situations and experiences which have some element of (often unconscious) fear.

Countertransference. The psychotherapist's emotional reaction, conscious and unconscious, to his patient and to the conflicts which the patient stimulates in the therapist.

Defense Mechanism/Defense. Any of a number of organized ways in which the ego or "self" protects itself from possible emotional danger, either from within (e.g., from dangerous impulses) or without (e.g., from threatening environmental situations). Defense mechanisms include conversion, repression, displacement, reaction formation, projection, isolation, identification, regression, introjection, and denial.

Delirium. A symptom of organic CNS disturbance characterized by confusion and altered consciousness.

Delusion. An inappropriate, false, unshakable belief (e.g., delusions of grandeur or persecution).

Dementia. Loss of intellectual ability due to organic CNS deficit.

Dependency Needs. Ubiquitous, but in adults usually repressed, needs for gratification from a parenting figure (e.g., love, security, food, warmth).

Depersonalization. A feeling that one is not oneself, that one's body is not one's own. Often includes the experience of "watching oneself" do things as if someone else were doing them.

Derealization. Similar to depersonalization, but a feeling that an environment which should be familiar is strange and without meaning.

Dereistic. Illogical, unrelated to reality.

Displacement. An unconscious defense mechanism in which feelings are transferred from a threatening object to one which can safely be used to deal with a conflict.

Dissociation. An unconscious defense mechanism in which feelings and affect are separated from the situation with which they are associated. Such an activity decreases the impact of the conflict on the ego (e.g., some forms of amnesia).

Double Bind. A situation, or form of interaction, in which an individual cannot choose between two alternatives without automatically contradicting his intent (e.g., a situation in which a child is criticized for being overweight but is made to feel guilty if he does not partake heartily of his mother's cooking).

Drive. A partially biological concept usually understood to represent the primitive wishes or impulses ("instincts") which supply both energy for and threat to the workings of the ego or self. Schematically, drives originate in the "id."

Ego. That portion of the emotional apparatus which mediates between the drives (see above), internalized prohibitions ("superego," "conscience"), and the external world. The ego shapes and transforms drive energy from the id into a more productive, less destructive form.

Ego-Dystonic/Ego-Syntonic. Connote the relationship of one's attitudes and behavior to one's total personality. Ego-dystonic behavior, for example, would be likely to cause anxiety or other discomfort, whereas ego-syntonic behavior would not.

Empathy. A subjective sharing and awareness of the feelings of another person.

Extrapyramidal Symptoms. Symptoms of CNS deficit in the extrapyramidal system, including the basal ganglia. These are frequently seen as reversible side effects of neuroleptic medications and include certain tremors, rigidity, akathisia, shuffling gait, some dysarthrias, and the like.

Extraversion. The directing of attention and activity outwardly from the self.

Fantasy. A series of imaginary images or events, such as daydreams but also including very brief flights of fancy, which express conflict and decrease emotional tension in an acceptable way (i.e., without action).

Fetish. An inanimate object which is given special symbolic meaning related to intrapsychic need or conflict. Sometimes an imperative part of sexual activity.

Fixation. A partial arrest of psychic development. Schematically, difficulties during a particular stage of development require that extra amounts of emotional energy remain invested at that stage, theoretically limiting energy available for future developmental and coping tasks. Under stress, an individual may "regress" to behavior which reflects this earlier level of defense.

Flight of Ideas. A skipping from one subject to another during conversation, which does not reflect continuous, logical thought process.

Folie à deux. The existence of the same, or complementary, delusions in two closely related persons.

Free Association. In psychoanalytic psychotherapy, the patient's continuous, uncensored expression of whatever thoughts or images come to mind.

Fugue. Severe dissociation of the personality from the environment. Often accompanied by amnesia or physical escape.

Functional. Often compared with "organic," "functional" disorders are those which are not attributable to known structural alterations. Psychogenic disorders are functional; however, not all functional disorders are psychogenic (e.g., a reaction to LSD). "Functional" does not imply "voluntary."

Gender. One's masculinity or femininity. "Gender identity" is culturally determined and is established very early in life. "Gender role" is the learned role which an individual assumes in order to perform as a male or female. "Sexual identity" refers to one's biological sex.

Gestalt. Refers to the total configuration of a whole (e.g., of an emotional situation) and the relationships among the parts of that whole.

Hallucination. A false sensory perception without external stimulus.

Hallucinosis. The state of hallucinating with clear consciousness (i.e., without delirium or other confusion).

Homosexual Panic. Acute, severe anxiety brought on by unconscious conflict related to issues of homosexuality. Does not connote overt homosexuality, nor does it require a sexual situation for precipitation.

Hysteria. Clinically, a condition of conversion of anxiety-producing conflict into a less threatening state (see "conversion"). Like other defensive mechanisms, a predominance of such symptoms may be described as an "hysterical neurosis." "Hysterical personality" is a chronic personality disorder which is manifested by emotional instability, attention seeking, theatrics, and overreaction, all often unconscious, accompanied by dependence and narcissism. "Hysterics" is a non-diagnostic lay term for uncontrolled emotional outbursts.

Id. The part of the personality which contains the unconscious impulses and drives. The id is the most primitive part of the personality. Its energies, in transmuted form, are used for the functions of the ego and superego.

Ideas of Reference. The delusion that external events refer directly to oneself (e.g., television newscasts, the arrangement of papers on a desk).

Identification. An unconscious defense mechanism in which the individual attempts or fantasizes becoming like someone else. The person who is the object of the identification may be either a threat or an ideal, or both.

Identity. A sense of "self" as a unique, stable entity which is basically unchanged by internal and external events. An "identity crisis," commonly seen in adolescents, refers to the anxiety which is felt when one seriously questions one's identity, either on a personal or philosophical basis.

Illusion. An erroneous interpretation of real sensory input.

Impulse. In psychoanalysis, a primitive drive or instinct. "Impulse disorders" are those in which one's control over impulses is weak, resulting in ego-syntonic impulsive behavior.

Incorporation. An unconscious defense mechanism in which a representation of some other person (or some attribute of the other person) is "ingested" and becomes part of one's psychic environment. A form of introjection.

Infantile Sexuality. Describes a basic characteristic of early development and refers to the gratification of basic body needs, accompanied by pleasurable sensations which eventually become an end in themselves. Related to later sexual development but is by no means equivalent to the lay term "sexuality."

Instinct. An innate drive. Although not equivalent to animal "instincts," the term illustrates the interdependent relationship between biological substrate ("readiness") and subsequent emotional development.

Intellectualization. A defense mechanism in which intellectual exercise and reasoning defend against the surfacing of unconscious conflict.

Internalization. The ongoing process by which interactions between the individual and the external world are replaced by internal representations of these reactions and their results. Thus, a person with an overly strong conscience may be said to have a "punitive superego" related to conflicts involving the representations of one or both parents within the psyche.

Introjection.   An unconscious defense mechanism, closely related to internalization, in which objects which give rise to conflict are symbolically taken into the self. Less primitive than incorporation, since incorporation implies ingestion.

Introversion.   A turning inward of one's activities to the point of preoccupation with oneself and decreased interest in the external world.

Isolation.   An unconscious defense mechanism in which an unacceptable impulse, feeling, or act is separated from its source of conflict, thereby decreasing the emotional reaction (e.g., anxiety) associated with it.

Labile.   Unstable. Especially refers to inappropriate shifts of affect (e.g., from laughter to tears within a few moments).

Libido.   Broad term for emotional energy associated with drives for pleasurable gratification. The libido and its companion, aggressive drive energy, may be schematically considered to supply the raw energy for emotional ("psychosexual") development and behavior.

Magical Thinking.   Refers to the premise that one's thoughts are equivalent to action. Seen normally in children, dreams, rituals, and the like. Also seen abnormally in some psychiatric patients.

McNaghten Rule/M'Naghten Rule.   The earliest precedent in modern British and American law which, based upon one's mental status, modifies one's responsibility for crimes. Considerably modified or replaced in most jurisdictions by the Currens Formula, Durham Rules, and the concept of "irresistible impulse."

Narcissism. The directing or investment of libido inwardly toward oneself. Seen in normal self-esteem, as well as in self-centeredness and, more seriously, in psychoses in which the external world becomes completely unimportant.

Negativism. Severe resistance to outside suggestion or influence. Normal in some stages of infancy.

Neologism. Literally a "new word," generally meaningless but which may, when expressed by certain (e.g., schizophrenic) patients, be symbolic of complex ideas or conflicts.

Nervous Breakdown. A nonmedical, nondiagnostic lay term for mental disorder. When used in a medical context it should be clarified and made specific.

Neurosis/Psychoneurosis. An emotional means of adapting to the anxiety which is the result of unresolved, unconscious conflict. Neuroses involve defense mechanisms which prevent unacceptable ideas and feelings from reaching consciousness (see examples elsewhere in Glossary). Although all are considered psychiatrically maladaptive, examples of most defense mechanisms can be found in most people. From a practical point of view, the "normality" of neurotic traits or behaviors should always be related to the amount of discomfort or disability which they bring to the individual or those around him. Neither serious personality disorganization nor difficulty interpreting external reality is ordinarily seen in neuroses.

Nihilism. A delusion of, or behavior which suggests feelings of, nonexistence of the self or one of its parts.

Object. In psychiatry, a thing (usually a person) which can be the recipient or target of strong feelings ("cathexis"). "Object relations" refers to cathexis of or emotional involvement with an individual outside of oneself. "Object loss" refers to the actual or symbolic loss of a loved object (or the loss of the love itself), as through separation, illness, or death.

Obsession. Any thought which repeatedly and involuntarily intrudes on one's consciousness and cannot be eliminated by ordinary thinking. See "Compulsion."

Oedipus Complex/Oedipal Phase. A complicated dynamic process, extremely important to emotional development, which occurs in early childhood but which may not be completely resolved for many years (or ever). Applies to children of both sexes and involves the conscious and unconscious experiencing of attraction to the parent of the opposite sex, fear and aggression toward the parent of the same sex, and to a slightly lesser extent attraction for the parent of the same sex and fear and aggression toward the parent of the opposite sex. The many potential experiences and outcomes of these interactions contribute greatly to the form and extent of one's later neurotic adaptations to oneself and to the external environment.

Orthopsychiatry. An approach to mental disorders and human behavior which recognizes the combined efforts of the behavioral, medical, and social sciences, with emphasis on healthy emotional development and growth.

Overcompensation. Exaggerated correction of a real or imagined deficit (e.g., the disabled person who becomes an athlete despite the predictions of his doctors, *or* the person with feelings of inferiority who "conquers" them by becoming successful and powerful).

Overdetermination. Refers to the fact that psychiatric symptoms, feelings or behaviors are always related to a number of different, intersecting causal processes.

Paranoid. Refers to strong feelings, perhaps approaching delusional quality, of suspiciousness, jealousy, persecution, and/or grandeur.

Parapraxis. A slip or blunder, for example, a misspoken word or memory lapse. When examined psychiatrically, can be found to be symptomatic or symbolic and determined by unconscious motives.

Parapsychology. The study of events caused or perceived through some route other than physical cause and effect. The events are considered to be "real" and not manifestations of misperception or psychiatric disturbance.

Penis Envy. A condition symbolically related to the phallic phase of psychosexual development but more generally understood as the female wish for male characteristics or advantages.

Personality Disorder. One of several emotional disorders characterized by chronic, deeply ingrained patterns of behavior. Because of the chronicity and the severe effect on personality organization, these are considered different from neuroses and psychoses.

Perversion. A clinical term often erroneously used in a pejorative sense which describes any of a variety of sexual practices which deviate in either goal or object choice from culturally "normal" genital union. The term is properly used if the particular deviation represents a large proportion of one's total sexual activity.

Phobia. A persistent, obsessive fear of an object or situation which ordinarily would not be expected to elicit such strong affect. True phobias are the result of displacement of unconscious conflict onto external objects which are in some way symbolic of that conflict. "Traumatic phobias" also exist, such as in a child who is afraid of dogs after being bitten severely; however, phobic avoidance should not be confused with ordinary fear or "common sense."

Pleasure Principle. The Freudian concept that much of man's emotional development, unconscious adaptation, and behavior is based upon an instinctive striving for gratification and avoidance of discomfort. This concept is somewhat modified but not eliminated by the "reality principle," in which the requirements of the external world impinge upon one's internal drives.

Postpartum Psychosis/Postpartum Depression. An acute, severe emotional disturbance which may mimic schizophrenia or affective disorders and which follows childbirth. Possibly related to both emotional and organic (e.g., toxic) factors, this condition does not necessarily portend future serious psychiatric problems.

Preconscious. Refers to those thoughts which, although not in consciousness, can be readily brought into awareness by the focusing of one's attention upon them.

Primary Process. Both a noun and an adjective. Refers to unstructured, non-cause-and-effect mental activity characteristic of the unconscious mind. Ordinarily not a part of waking thought and communication except in some severely disturbed patients. See "secondary process."

Projection. An unconscious defense mechanism in which things which are emotionally unacceptable to oneself are (usually erroneously) attributed to and seen in others.

Psychodynamics. The area of study which recognizes the role of unconscious motivation (conflict, avoidance of anxiety, etc.) in behavior.

Psychoneurosis. See "neurosis."

Psychophysiologic/Psychosomatic. Refers to characteristics and/or disorders which reflect the interactions of the mind and body. In psychophysiologic disorders the emotions cause or affect disorders of a particular organ system (e.g., ulcers, asthma, some cardiac arrhythmias). Such effects are unconscious; "psychosomatic" should not be confused with "voluntary" or "malingering."

Psychosexual Development. A term which describes the observed process of emotional development from birth to maturity. Five "phases" are generally recognized:

Oral Phase: Birth to 12–18 months. Characterized by physical and emotional development which is, like the following phases, based upon the infant's biological characteristics and readiness. Thus, most experience, expression, and gratification are centered around the mouth and ingestion.

Anal Phase: Overlapping wtih the above, 1½–3 years. Experience, expression, and gratification are centered around the anus and elimination.

Phallic Phase: Overlaps with the above, 2½–6 years, sometimes called the Oedipal Phase. Experience, expression, and gratification center around the genitals and increasing awareness of sexual and gender identity.

Latency: Overlapping with the Phallic Phase, from about 6–12 years. Often erroneously considered to be a quiescent period of development, it is actually a time in which infantile sexual (developmental) activity and the energy related to it are displaced into socially approved areas (especially learning).

Genital Phase: The last stage of development. Overlaps with latency but generally starts with puberty. During this stage many of the issues of infantile development reemerge for more or less final resolution and the individual becomes capable of mature, reality-based functioning and lasting, appropriate object relations.

Psychosis. A term used to denote either a syndrome or a severe mental disorder which is associated with marked personality disorganization and regression. Such a condition may be related to organic and/or functional causes and is generally manifested by impairment of thinking, communication, behavior, and contact with reality which is so severe that it interferes with what are considered "appropriate" interactions with others and the external environment.

Psychotomimetic. Generally refers to certain drugs ("hallucinogens") which produce psychotic states or behaviors.

Rapport. A conscious feeling of mutual interaction and harmony between patient and therapist or physician. Often results in increased confidence and cooperation from the patient.

Rationalization. An unconscious defense mechanism in which an individual attempts to justify, sometimes in apparently plausible ways, conflictual feelings and behaviors.

Reaction Formation. An unconscious defense mechanism in which a particularly affect-laden impulse is controlled by means of attitudes and behaviors which are apparently opposite to it (e.g., strong, unacceptable sexual impulses which are transformed into strong attitudes against pornography).

Regression. A general term which describes both normal and abnormal real or symbolic returning to earlier (more "infantile") coping mechanisms.

Repression. An unconscious defense mechanism which prevents unacceptable impulses from reaching consciousness in recognizable form.

Resistance. In psychotherapy, the conscious and unconscious ways in which an individual defends against revelation (to himself) of unconscious material.

Secondary Process. Organized, cause-and-effect mental activity. It is characteristic of the ego and is the result of modification of primary process ("id") impulses and the effects of the external environment. The ordinary mode of thinking, communicating, and behaving in adult life.

Self-Image. The image which one has of oneself as the total of body image and emotional state. It may be conscious, unconscious, realistic, and/or inappropriate.

Separation Anxiety. In infants, fear and anxiety seen when the mother or parent figure is removed or when the child is approached by strangers. Symbolic remnants may appear later in life.

Sexual Deviation. See "perversion."

Sibling Rivalry. Competition between siblings for the love and attention (gratification) represented by the parent(s). May appear symbolically at other times in development and later in life.

Sublimation. An unconscious defense mechanism in which unacceptable drives and conflicts are diverted into acceptable channels.

Superego. A schematic representation of the part of the personality which is associated with morality and self-observation. The superego arises out of the young child's ego, is fueled by energy from the id, and is shaped by the internalization of an identification with the attitudes of parents and significant others in the child's environment. Similar to the concept of "conscience."

Suppression. A conscious effort (as opposed to the unconscious "repression") toward the control of unacceptable thoughts and impulses.

Symbol/Symbolism. In psychiatry, the representation of an external object as an intrapsychic concept (e.g., the young child may shape his behavior based upon feelings which are related to introjected representations of his parents). *Also,* the conscious representation, often disguised, of unconscious objects, impulses and conflicts.

Transference. The unconscious endowment of a person with feelings originally associated with some important other person(s) from one's early life. Although this phenomenon occurs to some extent in many interpersonal relationships, in psychotherapy it is readily seen when the patient begins to respond to feelings about the therapist which are based not upon the therapist's own characteristics, but upon exaggerated or fantasized similarities which the patient sees (unconsciously) between the therapist and, for example, the patient's mother or father.

Trauma. In psychiatry, a significant emotional experience which interferes with development or coping mechanisms. The stimulus may come from the external world or, in some instances, from the surfacing of overwhelming internal impulses. Although individual traumatic experiences are not, in and of themselves, felt to be sufficient to produce lasting neurotic adaptation, traumatic events are usually followed by regression, inhibition, and often physical symptoms.

Unconscious. Both an adjective and a noun, referring to that part of the mind whose content is not subject to awareness. Unconscious material is, however, of extreme importance in determining one's emotional functioning and behavior. The unconscious contains material which has never become conscious and material which has been conscious at some point in development but is now repressed and unavailable to the individual.

Undoing. An unconscious defense mechanism in which a conscious or unconscious unacceptable impulse or activity is symbolically acted out in reverse ("undone"). Like other defense mechanisms, undoing relieves anxiety but does not resolve the original conflict, and thus tends to be repeated over and over.

Waxy Flexibility/Cerea Flexibilitas.   A condition, sometimes present in catatonic patients, in which the seemingly rigid body can be manipulated by another person and will remain in the posture in which it is placed.

Word Salad.   A manifestation of severe looseness of associations in which an individual's words and phrases are seemingly random and without coherence.

Working Through.   In general, the exploration of a therapeutic issue, over time, by the patient with the help of the therapist. More specifically, work done by the patient, with the participation of the therapist, during which rejection of or resistance to insight is eventually transcended and lasting change (e.g., conviction based upon personal experience) is accomplished.

Bibliography

Anastasi, A. *Psychological Testing,* 4th Edition. New York: Macmillan, 1976.

Bourne, P. G. (Ed.): *Acute Drug Abuse Emergencies.* New York: Academic Press of Harcourt, Brace, Jovanovich, 1976.

Diagnostic and Statistical Manual—II. Committee on Nomenclature of the American Psychiatric Association, Washington, D.C., 1968.

Diagnostic and Statistical Manual—III. in preparation. Will supersede and modify the terminology in DSM—II.

Freedman, A. M., Kaplan, H. I., Sadock, B. J. (Eds.): *Comprehensive Textbook of Psychiatry—II.* Baltimore: Williams & Wilkins, 1975 (*Synopsis* of the above, with revisions, Williams & Wilkins, 1976).

Kaplan, H. S.: *The New Sex Therapy: Active Treatment of Sexual Dysfunctions.* New York: Brunner/Mazel, 1974.

Kubler-Ross, E.: *On Death and Dying.* New York: MacMillan, 1969.

Lipton, M. A., DiMascio, A., Killan, K. F. (Eds.): *Psychopharmacology: A Generation of Progress.* New York: Raven Press, 1978.

Nicholi, A. M., Jr. (Ed): *The Harvard Guide to Modern Psychiatry.* Cambridge, MA: Belknap Press of Harvard University Press, 1978.

Shader, R. I. (Ed.): *Manual of Psychiatric Therapeutics.* Boston: Little, Brown, 1975.

Steinhauer, P. D., Rae-Grant, Q. (Eds.): *Psychological Problems of the Child and His Family.* Toronto: Macmillan of Canada, 1977.

Verwoerdt, A.: *Clinical Geropsychiatry.* Baltimore: Williams & Wilkins, 1976.

Werry, J. S. (Ed.): *Pediatric Psychopharmacology: The Use of Behavior Modifying Drugs in Children.* New York: Brunner/Mazel, 1978.

Wittkower, E. D., Warnes, H. (Eds.): *Psychosomatic Medicine: Its Clinical Applications.* Hagerstown, MD: Medical Department, Harper & Row, 1977.